DIGITAL TECHNIQUES IN ECHOCARDIOGRAPHY

DEVELOPMENTS IN CARDIOVASCULAR MEDICINE

Recent volumes

Hanrath P, Bleifeld W, Souquet, J. eds: Cardiovascular diagnosis by ultrasound. Transesophageal, computerized, contrast, Doppler echocardiography. 1982. ISBN 90-247-2692-1.

Roelandt J, ed: The practice of M-mode and two-dimensional echocardiography. 1983. ISBN 90-247-2745-6.

Meyer J, Schweizer P, Erbel R, eds: Advances in noninvasive cardiology. 1983. ISBN 0-89838-576-8.

Morganroth J, Moore EN, eds: Sudden cardiac death and congestive heart failure: Diagnosis and treatment. 1983. ISBN 0-89838-580-6.

Perry HM, ed: Lifelong management of hypertension. 1983. ISBN 0-89838-582-2.

Jaffe EA, ed: Biology of endothelial cells. 1984. ISBN 0-89838-587-3.

Surawicz B, Reddy CP, Prystowsky EN, eds: Tachycardias. 1984. ISBN 0-89838-588-1.

Spencer MP, ed: Cardiac Doppler diagnosis. 1983. ISBN 0-89838-591-1.

Villarreal H, Sambhi MP, eds: Topics in pathophysiology of hypertension. 1984. ISBN 0-89838-595-4.

Messerli FH, ed: Cardiovascular disease in the elderly. 1984. ISBN 0-89838-596-2.

Simoons ML, Reiber JHC, eds: Nuclear imaging in clinical cardiology. 1984. ISBN 0-89838-599-7.

Ter Keurs HEDJ, Schipperheyn JJ, eds: Cardiac left ventricular hypertrophy. 1983. ISBN 0-89838-612-8.

Sperelakis N, ed: Physiology and pathophysiology of the heart. 1984. ISBN 0-89838-615-2.

Messerli FH, ed: Kidney in essential hypertension. 1984. ISBN 0-89838-616-0.

Sambhi MP, ed: Fundamental fault in hypertension. 1984. ISBN 0-89838-638-1.

Marchesi C, ed: Ambulatory monitoring: Cardiovascular system and allied applications. 1984. ISBN 0-89838-642-X.

Kupper W, MacAlpin RN, Bleifeld W, eds: Coronary tone in ischemic heart disease. 1984. ISBN 0-89838-646-2.

Sperelakis N, Caulfield JB, eds: Calcium antagonists: Mechanisms of action on cardiac muscle and vascular smooth muscle. 1984. ISBN 0-89838-655-1.

Godfraind T, Herman AS, Wellens D, eds: Calcium entry blockers in cardiovascular and cerebral dysfunctions. 1984. ISBN 0-89838-658-6.

Morganroth J, Moore EN, eds: Interventions in the acute phase of myocardial infarction. 1984. ISBN 0-89838-659-4.

Abel FL, Newman WH, eds: Functional aspects of the normal, hypertrophied, and failing heart. 1984. ISBN 0-89838-665-9.

Sideman S, Beyar R, eds: Simulation and imaging of the cardiac system. 1985. ISBN 0-89838-687-X.

Van der Wall E, Lie KI, eds: Recent views on hypertrophic cardiomyopathy. 1985. ISBN 0-89838-694-2.

Beamish RE, Singal PK, Dhalla NS, eds: Stress and heart disease. 1985. ISBN 0-89838-709-4.

Beamish RE, Panagio V, Dhalla NS, eds: Pathogenesis of stress-induced heart disease. 1985. ISBN 0-89838-710-8.

Morganroth J, Moore EN, eds: Cardiac arrhythmias. 1985. ISBN 0-89838-716-7.

Mathes E, ed: Secondary prevention in coronary artery disease and myocardial infarction. 1985. ISBN 0-89838-736-1.

Lowell Stone H, Weglicki WB, eds: Pathology of cardiovascular injury. 1985. ISBN 0-89838-743-4.

Meyer J, Erbel R, Rupprecht HJ, eds: Improvement of myocardial perfusion. 1985. ISBN 0-89838-748-5.

Reiber JHC, Serruys PW, Slager CJ: Quantitative coronary and left ventricular cineangiography. 1986. ISBN 0-89838-760-4.

Fagard RH, Bekaert IE, eds: Sports cardiology. 1986. ISBN 0-89838-782-5.

Reiber JHC, Serruys PW, eds: State of the art in quantitative coronary arteriography. 1986. ISBN 0-89838-804-X.

Roelandt J, ed: Color Doppler Flow Imaging. 1986. ISBN 0-89838-806-6.

Van der Wall EE, ed: Noninvasive imaging of cardiac metabolism. 1986. ISBN 0-89838-812-0.

Liebman J, Plonsey R, Rudy Y, eds: Pediatric and fundamental electrocardiography. 1986. ISBN 0-89838-815-5.

Hilger HH, Hombach V, Rashkind WJ, eds: Invasive cardiovascular therapy. 1987. ISBN 0-89838-818-X

Serruys PW, Meester GT, eds: Coronary angioplasty: a controlled model for ischemia. 1986. ISBN 0-89838-819-8.

Tooke JE, Smaje LH: Clinical investigation of the microcirculation. 1986. ISBN 0-89838-819-8.

Van Dam RTh, Van Oosterom A, eds: Electrocardiographic body surface mapping. 1986. ISBN 0-89838-834-1.

Spencer MP, ed: Ultrasonic diagnosis of cerebrovascular disease. 1987. ISBN 0-89838-836-8.

Legato MJ, ed: The stressed heart. 1987. ISBN 0-89838-849-X.

Roelandt J, ed: Digital techniques in echocardiography. 1987. ISBN 0-89838-861-9.

Sideman S, Beyar R, eds: Activation, metabolism and perfusion of the heart. 1987. ISBN 0-89838-871-6.

DIGITAL TECHNIQUES IN ECHOCARDIOGRAPHY

edited by

J. ROELANDT
Thoraxcenter, Erasmus University,
Rotterdam, The Netherlands

1987 **MARTINUS NIJHOFF PUBLISHERS**
a member of the KLUWER ACADEMIC PUBLISHERS GROUP
DORDRECHT / BOSTON / LANCASTER

Distributors

for the United States and Canada: Kluwer Academic Publishers, P.O. Box 358, Accord Station, Hingham, MA 02018-0358, USA
for the UK and Ireland: Kluwer Academic Publishers, MTP Press Limited, Falcon House, Queen Square, Lancaster LA1 1RN, UK
for all other countries: Kluwer Academic Publishers Group, Distribution Center, P.O. Box 322, 3300 AH Dordrecht, The Netherlands

Library of Congress Cataloging in Publication Data

```
Digital techniques in echocardiography.

   (Developments in cardiovascular medicine)
   Includes bibliographies and index.
   1. Ultrasonic cardiography--Digital techniques.
2. Contrast echocardiography--Digital techniques.
I. Roelandt, Jos.  II. Series.  [DNLM: 1. Echocardio-
graphy--methods.  2. Heart--radionuclide imaging.
W1 DE997VME / WG 141.5.E2 D572]
RC683.5.U5D54  1987    616.1'207543      86-33217
ISBN 0-89838-861-9 (U.S.)
```

ISBN 0-89838-861-9

PRINTED IN THE NETHERLANDS

Table of Contents

VI

Preface

Cardiac ultrasound has rapidly developed into one of the most important clinical methods for diagnosis and follow-up of patients with heart disease and has changed the practice of cardiology permanently. In addition to improving image quality, most of the progress relies on digital image acquisition, storage, and quantitative analysis equipment. Automatic endocardial detection and three-dimensional reconstruction are now being developed. The progress with contrast echocardiography for myocardial perfusion imaging and results with tissue characterization is slow, but ever increasing, illustrating that the full potential of the method has not yet been explored. All of these digital techniques are extensively dealt with in this volume. Computerized tools will help the clinical cardiologists in their daily practice and stimulate further development to genuinely improve patient care in the coming years.

We wish to thank the authors to this volume for their excellent contribution and Mrs. T. van der Kolk for secretarial assistance.

Contributors

F.J. ten Cate
  Thorax Center, Erasmus University, P.O. Box 1738, 3000 DR Rotterdam, The
  Netherlands
R. Erbel
  II Medical Clinic, Johannes Gutenberg University, Langenbeckstr. 1, P.O.
  Box 3960, D-6500 Mainz, FRG
    Co-authors: R. Zotz, B. Henkel, G. Schreiner, C. Steuernagel, R. Zahn,
    H. Kopp, W. Clas, R. Brennecke, P. Schweizer, J. Meyer
S.B. Feinstein
  Division of Cardiology, Box 44, University of Chicago, 950 East 59th Street,
  Chicago, IL 60637, USA
D.G. Gibson
  Department of Cardiology, Brompton Hospital, Fulham Road, London SW3
  6HP, UK
    Co-author: R.B. Logan Sinclair
E. Grube
  Medical University Clinic, Cardiology-Internal Medicine, Sigmund Freudstr.
  25, D-5300 Bonn 1, FRG
    Co-authors: H. Becher & B. Backs (Cand. Inform., Königstrasse 25, D-5300
    Bonn 1, FRG)
R.J.C. Hall
  Cardiology Department, Royal Victoria Infirmary, Queen Victoria Road,
  Newcastle upon Tyne, NE1 4LP, UK
R.H. Hoyt
  Department of Internal Medicine, University of Arizona Health Sciences
  Center, Tucson, AZ 85724, USA
    Co-authors: S.M. Collins & D.J. Skorton; Dept of Internal Medicine,
    University of Iowa, Iowa City, IA 52242, USA
J.A. Kisslo
  Department of Medicine, Duke University, P.O. Box 3818, Durham, NC
  27710, USA

Co-authors: J.E. Snyder & O.T. von Ramm (Biomedical Engineering, Duke University, Durham, NC 27710, USA

R.S. Meltzer
Cardiology Division, Mount Sinai Medical Center, One Gustave Levy Pl., New York, NY 10029, USA

S.M. Powsner
Division of Cardiology, Box 44, University of Chicago, 950 East 59th Street, Chicago, IL 60637, USA
Co-author: S.B. Feinstein

Part One: Contrast Echocardiography

1. Developments in Echo Contrast Agents

Steven B. FEINSTEIN
University of Chicago, USA

Introduction

Contrast echo techniques are beginning to be used to assess blood flow within the myocardial tissue of man, and progress to date suggests that, with further development, contrast echo may fulfill the critical clinical need to quantitate myocardial perfusion and actual tissue at risk [1, 2, 3]. The ability to quantitate perfusion and define at-risk tissue would be particularly timely due to the recent advances made in salvaging viable myocardial tissue using such techniques as thrombolysis, angioplasty, early surgical revascularization and, potentially, laser therapy; generally, these techniques are currently performed based upon angiographic data, although recent reports describe the discrepancy between coronary artery anatomy as defined by the angiogram and the actual functional parameters of myocardial blood flow [4]. Optimally, the ideal imaging modality used to assess viable tissue would be one that is a functional parameter and is accurate, quantitative, readily available, non-invasive, non-toxic and economical.

Several centers around the world have performed early contrast echo studies, safely, in a variety of patient populations in order to provide the data necessary to evaluate myocardial viability. Santoso [5], Goldman [6, 7], and Feinstein [8] have demonstrated the feasibility of performing left heart intracoronary injections of small volumes of well-controlled microbubble solutions. In addition, significant advances in the field have led to the development of echo contrast agents that can readily pass through the lung capillaries and enter the myocardial tissue after an initial peripheral vein injection [9].

As a necessary criteria to this new technology, quantitative analyses must be performed on the microbubble backscatter relationship in order to quantitate perfusion. As a first step in quantifying echo contrast effects, a mathematical relationship has been demonstrated between microbubble size and concentration with that of radiofrequency backscatter analysis [10]. In addition, coronary and renal artery electromagnetic determinations, under varying blood conditions, have demonstrated that there exists a relationship between echo contrast disappearance time and blood flow [11, 12].

J. Roelandt (editor), Digital Techniques in Echocardiography. ISBN 0-89838-861-9.
© 1987, Martinus Nijhoff Publishers, Dordrecht. Printed in the Netherlands.

Ultimately, it may be possible to evaluate quantitatively the actual myocardial blood flow, using a single peripheral intravenous echo contrast agent injection and simultaneously performing an otherwise-conventional echocardiogram.

Historical development of echo contrast agents

Gramiak and Shah in 1968 first reported on the use of 'microbubble agents' for the purpose of enhancing the ultrasound image [13]. Their early studies were performed in the catheterization laboratory where, using freshly prepared Indocyanine Green, the aortic root flush revealed an intense echo image corresponding to the injection of the dye. Subsequently, several investigators at Rochester and elsewhere discovered that hydraulic cavitation process created small gaseous disruptions in the blood stream that were seen as echo contrast effects [14, 15] It was felt that the microbubbles created in these solutions were responsible for the contrast effects due to marked acoustic impedance [16].

Subsequently, contrast echo techniques used hand-agitated microbubbles for studies of valvular regurgitation [17, 18, 19], intracardiac shunts [20] and chamber identification [21].

Contrast echo techniques have become an alternative choice to X-ray angiography where a patient has a clinically significant medical problem such as severe congestive heart failure, renal disease, or other conditions that might endanger the patient's health if subjected to the dye load or radiation required. In addition, during pregnancy, contrast echo has been used to reduce the radiation exposure of standard angiography [22].

Investigators have used solutions of hand-agitated microbubbles to identify myocardial tissue perfusion in the experimental animal setting [23–28] as well as in man [5–7]. These early studies relied entirely upon the production of microbubbles from manual agitation. However, the possibility that these microbubbles tend to occlude capillary flow, rather than pass through as the red blood cells, has been investigated. Several independent studies using direct microscopic examination have demonstrated that these hand-agitated microbubbles were too large to pass through the capillaries in the same fashion as the red blood cells [29, 30].

Despite the non-physiologic myocardial transit times noted in the capillary circulation of these hand-agitated bubbles, several investigators have shown a correlation with the degree of coronary blood flow and contrast echo washout [31]. These experimental studies, taken together, have promoted the use of echo contrast agents in identifying myocardial perfusion defects.

Based upon these promising results and the relative safety noted in performing these studies [5, 6, 32], several investigators have recently extended these animal studies to the human experience. In 1983, Santoso et al. [5] first reported on the use of a hand-agitated colloid solution to identify perfusion defects at the time of catheterization. Subsequently, Goldman and Mindich in 1984 [6, 7] reported similar findings using agitated cardioplegia at the time of open heart surgery to identify myocardial perfusion and valvular defects.

However, due to the clinical need to quantitate the amount of blood flow in a tissue, the microbubble echo constant agents needed to be further refined in order to develop agents that are: (1) smaller than red blood cells (so as to flow unimpeded through the circulation, thus representing actual blood flow patterns within the myocardium), (2) stable, (3) persistent, (4) simple to prepare and (5) feasible for intravascular injections.

In 1982, Feinstein [33] first reported upon the use of a mechanical method (ultrasonic cavitation or sonication) to produce microbubbles that were smaller than red blood cells, safe, and stable enough to pass through the micro-vasculature of dogs. The solutions that were initially tested included Renografin-76, dextrose 50%, dextrose 70%, sorbitol 70%, Indocyanine Green, and saline. After the in vitro tests were completed [34], these sonicated solutions were tested against the hand-agitated solutions in the mesentery circulation system of a cat [30]. Consistent with prior reports, the smaller, more stable sonicated microbubbles of sorbitol 70% and dextrose 70%, readily passed through the capillaries, whereas the larger more unstable hand-agitated microbubbles tended to transiently occlude the circulation [29] (Figure 1). Subsequently, coronary artery, aortic root and renal injections in experimental animals revealed that the transit times through the tissue were affected by microbubble diameter [11, 12] (Table 1). Further studies demonstrated that only the small, stable sonicated microbubbles

Table 1. This table represents the microbubble diameter measurements (light microscopy and laser analysis) and the calculated myocardial video-intensity decay from a series of aortic root and intracoronary injections. The smallest bubbles found in solutions of either sonicated sorbitol or Renografin-76 consistently produce the most rapid video-intensity decay within the myocardial tissue, whereas, the larger more variable bubbles of dextrose 50% or 70% produce the longest video-intensity decay times.

MICROBUBBLE SIZE AND TRANSIT TIME

AGENT (sonicated)	DIAMETER(microns) microscope	laser	TRANSIT TIME (seconds) aortic root	intracoronary
Sorbitol 70%	6±2	2.0±1.5	2.3±1.2	6.0±2.0
Renografin-76	10±3	4.5±2.8	3.4±1.7	–
Dextrose 70%	8±3	4.6±2.8	5.1±2.0	11.4±4.6
Dextrose 50%	12±4	5.1±3.6	6.8±1.7	13.9±5.0

6

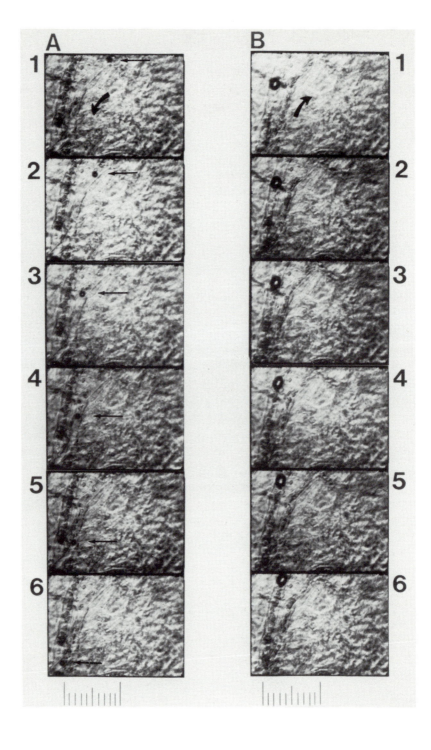

could successfully pass through the lungs, whereas, the larger hand-agitated microbubbles failed transpulmonary passage [35].

In order for the sonicated agents to become clinically useful in quantifying blood flow, two further questions must be addressed: (1) Do the microbubbles and blood flow rates correlate? and (2) What relationship exists between radio-frequency backscatter and the microbubbles?

Using a direct radiofrequency analysis of microbubble concentrations and backscatter relationships, Powsner [10] developed an in vitro model to test the mathematical formulations based upon Lord Rayleigh's sound wave scatter theories [36]. Using sonicated sorbitol microbubbles, a hemocytometer, an ultrasound transceiver, and an oscilloscope, Powsner demonstrated that, in fact, a mathematical relationship does exist between the radiofrequency backscatter, attenuation, diameter and concentration of the bubbles. [See also the chapter on Quantitation of Echo Contrast Effects.]

The blood flow and microbubble flow relationship was investigated in studies using electromagnetic flow meters placed on the coronary and renal arteries. Subsequently, direct aortic root, coronary artery, and renal artery injections revealed that the smallest sonicated bubbles (sorbitol 70%) pass readily through the microcirculation, whereas, other sonicated solutions pass quickly through the myocardium but small variations in microbubble diameters result in a consistent (albeit small) delay in blood flow transit times (see Table 1). These studies demonstrate that tissue transit calculations depend upon selecting the echo contrast agent that does not impede capillary flow.

Studies performed in the kidney have similarly cast light upon the relationship between sonicated microbubbles and blood flow. In these experiments, an electromagnetic flow probe was placed around the proximal portion of the renal artery, the kidney was directly exposed from a surgical incision and then was ultrasonically scanned. One milliliter of sonicated microbubbles of Renografin-76 was injected into the descending aorta. By direct, local infusion of either bradykinin or norepinephrine in the renal artery, the renal blood flow was altered and measured by electromagnetic flow probes. Correlations of renal blood flow and contrast echo disappearance rates by videodensity revealed a direct relationship. From these studies, there appears to be sufficient scientific evidence to support the contention that contrast ultrasonography may be a useful method to image blood flow in tissue.

←

Fig. 1. Composite photomicrographs of an intact cat capillary system illustrating the transit of microbubbles within the vasculature. Note the sequence on the left (A) reveals the unimpeded capillary passage of sonicated sorbitol microbubbles (light microscopy, diameter 6 ± 2 microns), whereas, the sequence on the right (B), the larger microbubbles of hand agitated Renografin-76 and saline (light microscopy 16 ± 13 microns) demonstrate transient vascular occlusion. The measurement grid is calibrated in 10 micron increments. This figure is reprinted with permission from the American College of Cardiology (Journal of the American College of Cardiology 1984; Volume 4, no. 3, page 597, figure 2(A) and (B)).

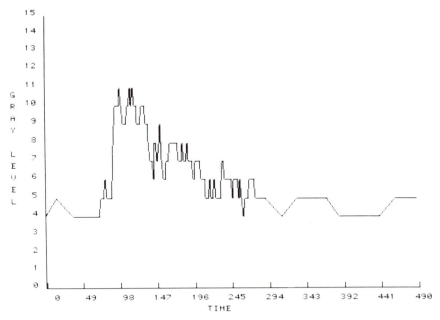

Fig. 2. This off-line computer-derived video density curve characterizes the ultrasound contrast appearance within a specific region of the myocardium. The pixel intensity is on the ordinate, and the time (frames per second) is on the abscissa. Note the characteristic pattern of baseline intensity, followed by a brisk rise (contrast injection) and the ultimate decay in intensity.*

Clinical studies

Contrast echo techniques dating back to 1968 have generally been used to identify valvular regurgitation [13, 17, 18, 19, 21], intracardiac shunts [20], and cardiac anatomy where radiation cannot be used [24]. Generally, the contrast techniques have been used as alternatives rather than primary diagnostic aids. Recent experimental studies defining myocardial perfusion in both the experimental [23–28] and clinical [5–8] settings have sparked renewed interest in using contrast echo techniques to define myocardial tissue viability.

At the University of Chicago, patients with normal or diseased coronary vessels and several patients undergoing percutaneous transluminal coronary angioplasty (PTCA) have been studied using direct intracoronary contrast agents (sonicated Renografin-76). To date, there have been no complications related to the contrast echo technique. In studies designed to quantitate the contractility effects of sonicated agents, no direct additive effects on contractility were noted due to the presence of microbubbles in both experimental and clinical studies. However, the carrier solutions (Renografin-76, dextrose 70, 50% and sorbitol 70%) all had varying effects on contractibility even without the addition of microbubbles [37].

* The figure is reprinted with permission from the American Journal of Cardiac Imaging 1987; Vol. 1, no. 1, p. 36, fig. 6.

9

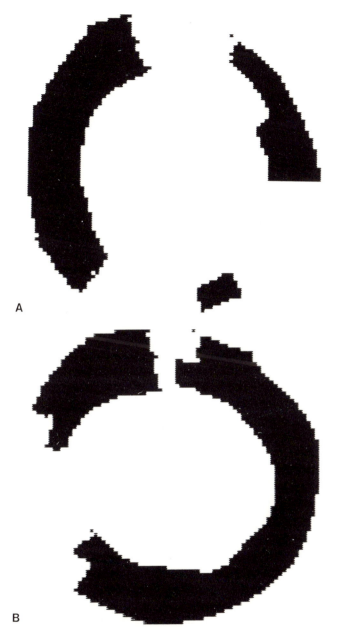

A

B

Fig. 3. The time and intensity of the videodensito metric analysis is represented in a single cross-sectional parametric image. These computer derived images were taken from a 42 year old patient undergoing elective coronary angiography. There was no evidence of significant coronary disease. The image on the left represents the spatial distribution of myocardial blood flow obtained from the right coronary system; the graph on the right represents the left coronary artery distribution. Note that there is a small area of overlap in the perfusion distribution.

The figure is reprinted with permission from the American Journal of Cardiac Imaging 1987; Vol. 1, no. 1, p. 34, fig. 4 (A) and (B).

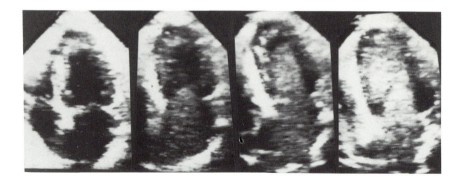

Fig. 4. These segmental photographs of a two-dimensional echocardiogram showing an apical 4 chamber view from an 18 kilogram monkey reveal the successful passage of sonicated albumin microspheres (2 to 4 microns in diameter) from right heart structures through to the left heart chambers. The first frame shows the baseline apical four chamber view with the right heart structures on the left and the left atrium and ventricle on the right. Following a peripheral arm vein injection of 3 ml of sonicated albumin microspheres, note the early echodense appearance of the microspheres in the right atrium. Shortly afterward, the bubbles now appear in the left atrium, having successfully passed through the lungs. The final photograph demonstrates the dense appearance of the micro-spheres within the left heart cavity. Subsequent histologic sections of the lungs, heart, kidney and liver failed to reveal evidence of hemorrhage or embolization.

These clinical studies have been analyzed by visual interpretation as well as by computer assisted videodensity measurements and subsequent correlations have been applied to the angiographically described coronary arteries. The regional perfusion areas and myocardial transit time (or $T^{1/}_{2}$) have been calculated for the intracoronary injections of sonicated Renografin-76 in patients (see Figures 2 and 3). Ultimately, the ability to define perfusion defects as well as quantitate regional myocardial blood flow based on varying degrees of coronary artery stenosis may, in fact, become a clinical technique.

Future prospects

Recently, our laboratory at the University of Chicago has developed echo contrast agents that are capable of transpulmonary passage resulting in myocardial perfusion identification from a single small peripheral vein injection. Sonicated air-filled albumin spheres ranging from 2 to 9 microns (with a mode of 2 to 4 microns) appear to be echogenic and stable for days. These agents have been tested in a variety of animals, and with a successful capillary passage of contrast material in each experiment. The figure [4] demonstrates the sequence of a peripheral forearm vein injection of 3 ml in an 18 kilogram rhesus monkey. Subsequent offline computer videodensity analysis revealed myocardial tissue intensity alteration due to the transit of the spheres through the myocardial tissue.

If, in fact, these transpulmonary agents can be stabilized for significant periods of time, and prove to be safe and efficacious, complete tissue perfusion data could ultimately be performed from a single vein injection using ultrasound. Beyond the scope of cardiology, the wider applications would include other organ systems such as: kidney, liver, and vascular tree.

Considering the advances made in interventional cardiology, and the need to identify viable tissue, contrast echo techniques appear to be an area of interest with considerable potential which may ultimately play an important role in the clinical diagnosis and management of patients with ischemic heart disease.

References

1. Skorton DJ, Collins SM: New Directions in Cardiac Imaging. Ann Int Med 1985; 102: 795–9.
2. Laffel GL, Braunwald E: Thrombolytic therapy, a new strategy for the treatment of acute myocardial infarction. NEJM 1984; 311: 770–6.
3. Vogel RA: The radiographic assessment of coronary blood flow parameters. CIRC 1984; 72(3) 460–5.
4. White CW, Creighton WB, Doty DB, Hiratza LF, Eastham CL, Harrison DG, Marcks ML: Does visual interpretation of the coronary angiogram predict the physiologic importance of a coronary stenosis? NEJM 1984; 310: 819–24.
5. Santoso T, Wiratmo B, Mansyur H, Rahman AM, Panggabean M, Abduraham N: Myocardial perfusion imaging in humans by contrast echocardiography using polygelin colloid solution. JACC 1985; 6(3): 612–20.
6. Goldman ME, Mindich BP: Intraoperative cardioplegia contrast echocardiography for assessing myocardial perfusion during heart surgery. JACC 1984; 4: 1029–34.
7. Goldman ME, Mindich BP: Intraoperative contrast echocardiography to evaluate mitral valve operations. JACC 1984; 4: 1035–40.
8. Feinstein SB, Lang RM, Neumann A, Al-Sadir J, Chua KG, Carroll JD, Keller MW, Powsner SM, Borow KM: Intracoronary contrast echocardiography in humans: perfusion and anatomic correlates. CIRC 1985; III–57 (abstract).
9. Keller MW, Feinstein SB; work in progress.
10. Powsner SM, Feinstein SB, Saniie J: Quantitative radiofrequency analysis of sonicated echo contrast agents. JACC 1985; 5: 474 (abstract).
11. Feinstein SB, Ong K, Shah PM, Staniloff H, Fujiyabasha Y, Zwehl W, Meerbaum S, Corday E: A new standardized, reproducible method for assessing regional myocardial blood flow with sonicated echo contrast agents. Circulation 1984; 70(Suppl II): II–4 (abstract).
12. Frederickson ED, McCoy CE, Powsner SM, Lang RM, Goldberg LI, Feinstein SB: Distribution of renal cortical blood flow measured by contrast ultrasonography. Clinical Res 1985; 33(2): 483A.
13. Gramiak R, Shah PM: Echocardiography of the aortic root. Invest Radiol 1968; 3: 356–66.
14. Ziskin MC, Bonakdarpour A, Weinstein DP, Lynch PR: Contrast agents for diagnostic ultrasound. Invest Radiol 1972; 7:500–5.
15. Kremkau FW, Gramiak R, Carstensen EL, Shah PM, Kramer H: Ultrasonic detection of cavitation at catheter tips. Am J Roentgenology 1970; 110: 177–83.
16. Meltzer RS, Tickner EG, Sahines TP: The source of ultrasound contrast effect. J Clin Ultrasound 1980; 8: 121–7.

12

17. Kerber RE, Kioschos JM, Lauer RM: Use of an ultrasonic contrast method in th diagnosis of valvular regurgitation and intracardiac shunts. Am J Cardio 1974; 34: 722–7.
18. Reid CL, Kawanishi DT, McKay CR, Elkayam U, Rahimtoola SH, Chanraratna PAN: Accuracy of evaluation of the presence and severity of aortic and mitral regurgitation by contrast 2-dimensional echocardiography. Am J Cardiol 1983; 52: 519.
19. Williams KA, Feinstein SB, Neumann A, Caroll JD, Frier PAS, Kremseu CB, Al-Sadir J, Chua KG, Borow KM: Microbubble contrast echocardiography for the assessment of valvular regurgitation: Comparison with cineangiography and Doppler echocardiography. Clin Res 1985; 33(2): 238A.
20. Sahn DJ, Valdez-Cruz LM: Ultrasonic contrast studies for the detection of cardiac shunts. JACC 1984; 3: 978–85.
21. Roelandt J: Contrast echocardiography. J Ultrasound in Med and Biol 1982; 8: 471.
22. Elkayam U, Kawanishi D, Reid CL, Chandraratna PAN, Gleicher N, Rahimtoola SH: Contrast echocardiography to reduce ionizing radiation associated with cardiac catheterization during pregnancy. Am J Cardiol 1983; 52: 213–4.
23. Tei C, Sakamaki T, Shah PM, Meerbaum S, Shimoura K, Kondo S, Corday E: Myocardial contrast echocardiography. Circulation 1982; 66: 166–74.
24. Armstrong W, Mueller T, Kinney E, Tickner G, Dillon J, Feigenbaum H: Assessment of myocardial perfusion abnormalities with contrast enhanced two-dimensional echocardiography. Circulation 1982; 66: 166–73.
25. Ten Cate FJ, Drury JK, Meerbaum S, Noordsy J, Feinstein S, Shah PM, Corday E: Myocardial contrast two-dimensional echocardiography: Experimental examination at different coronary flow levels. JACC 1984; 69: 418–29.
26. Kemper AJ, O'Boyle JE, Cohen CA, Taylor A, Parisi AF: Hydrogen peroxide contrast echocardiography: Quantification in vivo of myocardial risk area during coronary occlusion and of the necrotic area remaining after myocardial reperfusion. Circulation 1984; 70: 309–17.
27. Gaffney FA, Lin JC, Peshock RM, et al: Hydrogen peroxide contrast echocardiography. Am J Cardiol 1983; 52: 607.
28. Meltzer RS, Vermeulen HJ, Valk NK, Verdoux PD, Lancee CT, Roelandt J: New echocardiographic contrast agents: Transmission through the lungs and myocardial perfusion imaging. J Cardiovascular Ultrasonography 1982; 1: 277–82.
29. Kort A, Kronzon I: Microbubble formation: In vitro and in vivo observations. JCU 1982; 10: 117–20.
30. Feinstein SB, Shah PM, Bing RJ, Meerbaum S, Corday E, Chang B, Santillan G. Fujibayashi Y: Microbubble dynamics visualized in the intact capillary circulation. JACC 1984; 4: 595–600.
31. Tei C, Kondo S, Meerbaum S, Ong K, Maurer G, Wood F, Sakamaki T, Shimoura K, Corday E, Shah PM: Correlation of myocardial echo contrast disappearance rate ('washout') and severity of experimental coronary stenosis. JACC 1984; 3: 39–46.
32. Gillam LD, Kaul S, Fallon JT, Hedley-Whyte ET, Slater CE, Weyman AE: Sequelae of echocardiographic contrast: Studies of myocardium, brain and kidney. Circulation 1984; 70: II–6 (abstract).
33. Feinstein SB, Maurer G, Tei C, Shah PM, Meerbaum S, Corday E: In vitro comparisons of echo contrast agents. CIRC 1982; 66(Suppl II): II–188.
34. Feinstein SB, Ten Cate FJ, Zwehl W, Ong K, Maurer G, Tei C, Shah PM, Meerbaum S, Corday E: Two-dimensional contrast echocardiography. I. In vitro development and quantitative analysis of echo contrast agents. JACC 1984; 3: 14–20.
35. Ten Cate FJ, Feinstein S, Zwehl W, Meerbaum S, Corday E, Fishbein M, Shah PM: Two-dimensional contrast echocardiography. II. Transpulmonary studies. JACC 1984; 3: 21–7.
36. Rayleigh JWS: *The Theory of Sound*, 2nd Ed (1945) Dover Publishers, p. 272.
37. Lang R, Borow KM, Neumann A, Feinstein SB: Echo contrast agents: Effect of sonicated microbubbles and carrier solutions on left ventricular contractility. CIRC 1985; III–58 (abstract).

2. Quantitative Radiofrequency Analysis of Sonicated Echo Contrast Agents

Seth M. POWSNER, M.D. and Steven B. FEINSTEIN
University of Chicago, USA

Introduction

Quantitative perfusion imaging is critically important for the evaluation and management of medical therapy. Sonicated microbubble echo contrast agents make ultrasound perfusion imaging a real, and potentially more economic, alternative to more conventional techniques (X-ray angiography, cine-CT, radioisotopes, and Magnetic Resonance). Sonicated microbubbles are excellent ultrasound reflectors and they flow unimpeded through the capillary circulation (because of their uniformly small size). This paper reviews the major issues in the ongoing development of quantitative echo contrast perfusion imaging.

Quantitative perfusion imaging is distinctly different from anatomic imaging. Conventional angiography identifies only varying degrees of apparent blockage. Actual blood flow is not measured and must be inferred. When angiography is used in conjunction with treatments such as angioplasty, little information is provided about actual tissue salvage. Alternatively, thallium isotope uptake studies provide only a qualitative assessment related to perfusion.

Each specialty has its own need for quantitative perfusion imaging. Cardiologists and cardiac surgeons need to evaluate the effect of various drug and vascular treatments on myocardial perfusion. Nephrologists, and internists treating hypertension, are critically concerned with the effect of their interventions on regional renal blood flow. Evaluation of peripheral perfusion is of concern to many.

Echo contrast techniques have potential advantages over other techniques being developed. Cine-CT (fast computed axial tomography), PET (positron emission tomography), and MRI (magnetic reasonance imaging) are currently being used to develop clinically useful perfusion images. However, ultrasound equipment is orders of magnitude less expensive than any of these techniques even if its cost were to double. Also, unlike the first two, no ionizing radiation is required. In addition, quantitative ultrasound equipment can be moved around the hospital or clinic to provide immediate evaluation of angioplastic and surgical intervention.

J. Roelandt (editor), Digital Techniques in Echocardiography. ISBN 0-89838-861-9.

14

Echo contrast review

The development of echo contrast agents dates back less than 20 years to the fortuitous observations of Gramiak and Shah [1]. Shortly thereafter, researchers recognized that the contrast effect observed was due to miniscule air bubbles [2, 3]. Subsequent clinical studies have assumed a qualitative, simplistic understanding of echo contrast effect in order to delineate intracardiac shunts, valve regurgitation [4, 5], and myocardial perfusion in experimental animal models [6–10]. Nonetheless, simple hand-agitated saline solutions are in regular clinical use for imaging cardiac abnormalities in newborns and other patients whose kidneys cannot tolerate X-ray contrast agents.

Careful studies of hand-agitated contrast agents (saline, Renografin) have demonstrated that the bubbles were large (16μ ± 16) compared to red blood cells and could be seen trapped in the capillary circulation [11]. Other agents developed shortly after the hand-agitated solutions share the same drawbacks, including various air-filled capsules and dilute hydrogen peroxide mixtures [10]. Despite the prolonged myocardial transit times caused by capillary trapping, a number of animal studies have been done [12–14] and some human studies [15, 16] confirming that the large bubbles flow into the perfused regions of tissue and not into ischemic areas. They also indicate a relative degree of safety.

Echo contrast effects have been observed with fluorocarbon solutions [17]. It has also been suggested that a large bolus of saline or serum will produce an observable change in ultrasound reflectance. However, neither approach appears near clinical aplication.

The development of sonication as a technique for producing uniformly small microbubbles (< 10μ, 11) marks a major step towards quantitative perfusion imaging. These red cell sized microbubbles demonstrate physiologic flow in heart [18], kidney [19], and mesentary [20]. They have been successfully used to demonstrate renal regional perfusion changes caused by pharmacologic interventions in animal experiments. Human studies under way have shown basic perfusion patterns expected from vascular anatomy and continue to demonstrate that the agents are safe [21].

Current work on new echo contrast agents has been oriented towards finding an agent which can both be injected intravenously and cross the lungs reliably. There has been some success even with transpulmonary microbubbles [22]. An albumin-based microbubble agent has been reported [23] and Schering has made preliminary reports of an agent without disclosing its nature [24]. Attempts also are being made to simplify contrast agent preparation by the clinician.

A reliable transpulmonary echo contrast agent would pave the way to outpatient evaluation of perfusion: myocardial, renal, etc. This would also be true if a reliable technique could be developed using intravenous radiopaque agents with cine-CT or corresponding tracers for isotope imaging, or MRI, or PET. All share some common problems due to injection bolus spreading. Each imaging technology also presents its own peculiar technical difficulties.

Echo contrast agent acoustics

The essence of any contrast agent is that it differs markedly from normal human blood. X-ray contrast agents are generally expected to be radiopaque, but air in the pneumoencephalogram functions by being less radiopaque. Similarly, current echo contrast agents are acoustically more reflective than blood, but acoustically 'darker' agents are conceivable. It may be possible to use bolus injections of crystaloid or colloid solutions in the future if ultrasound equipment becomes sufficiently sensitive to detect the change in acoustic reflectance due to a temporary drop in local blood cell concentration. Until then, the acoustics of echo contrast agents is essentially the acoustics of small gas bubbles. Small particulate agents can be treated like small bubbles, save for their different acoustic impedance.

A small gas bubble in water is a very effective acoustic reflector [25]. Though air is orders of magnitude less dense than water, it is the incompressible nature of water relative to air that dominates. Both differences are additive and effect a large impedance discontinuity. The fundamental formulas for wave reflection by a sphere are due Rayleigh [26, see Morse and Ingard, 27 for a more modern treatment and formulas used here].

Figure 1 depicts a plane wave coming from the left impinging on a small bubble in the center. The formula for the relative intensity of the reflected wave (assuming that the bubble radius is much less than the wave length) is shown underneath. For a microbubble of air in water, the reflected (more accurately, the scattered) wave is depicted by concentric circles propagating outward.

In Figure 1 and in later formulas, 'N' is concentration, 'V' is volume, 'K' is wave number, 'a' is bubble radius, '(r,θ)' is a point relative to the center of the volume in question, '$\varkappa$' and 'p' are the compressibility and density of the contrast agent ($_o$), and the gas in the bubble ($_n$). Intensity is 'I' either incident ($_i$) or scattered ($_s$). Cross section is denoted by 'Σ'. The velocity of sound in the medium (water/blood/tissue) is denoted by 'C'; an interval of time by $\triangle T$ delta.

For the simplest analysis of microbubble contrast agents, treat each bubble as a small mirror of scattering cross section Σ_s. A small volume filled with such an agent is depicted in Figure 2. The scattered intensity is proportional to bubble concentration and scattering cross section (Σ_s) considering only a small volume. Σ_s can be related to the formula in Figure 1 by integrating over the surface of the receiver.

Figure 3 shows the larger picture, an ultrasound examination of the heart as a typical clinical contrast study. Figure 4 shows the same situation, but focusing down on the particular volume and acoustic path of interest. The acoustic elements along the path have been simplified into transmission and reception geometry factors summarizing the performance of the transducer, a path attenuation factor lumping together the proximal anatomy not under consideration (a squared factor as it is traversed to and fro), and finally the backscatter ratio for the small volume of interest.

16

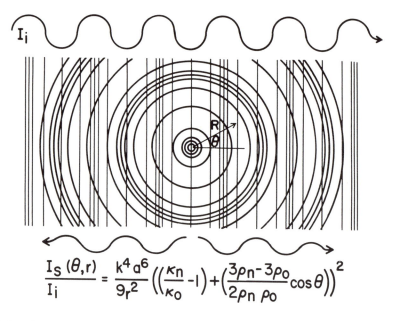

$$\frac{I_s\,(\theta,r)}{I_i} = \frac{k^4 a^6}{9r^2}\left(\left(\frac{\kappa_n}{\kappa_0}-1\right)+\left(\frac{3\rho_n-3\rho_0}{2\rho_n\,\rho_0}\cos\theta\right)\right)^2$$

Fig. 1. Rayleigh scattering by a microbubble (center) of a sound wave intensity I_i, (from left) resulting in a scattered wave (I_s). (r,θ) are coordinates relative to bubble, K is wave number, a is bubble radius, $\varkappa$ (Kappa) is compressability, ϱ (rho) is density, subscript $_0$ is for contrast agent, subscript $_n$ is for bubble gas.

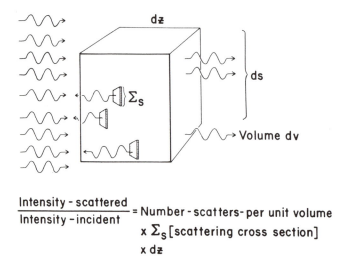

$$\frac{\text{Intensity - scattered}}{\text{Intensity - incident}} = \text{Number - scatters- per unit volume}$$
$$\times\ \Sigma_s\,[\text{scattering cross section}]$$
$$\times\ d\bar{z}$$

Fig. 2. Ultrasound scattering by microbubbles treated as a little mirrors with a small volume of interest (dv).

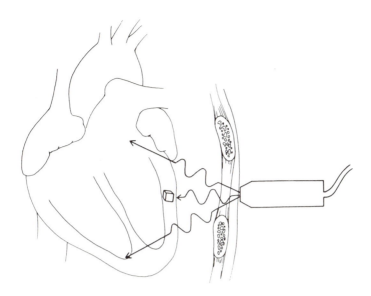

Fig. 3. Basic positioning of an ultrasound scanner's transducer (on right) to examine the human heart. Small cube represents a volume of specific interest.

The analysis in Figure 4 applies reasonably well only if the structures are stationary. For renal or hepatic studies this is approximately true. For cardiac studies it applies only during the transmission of a single pulse of ultrasound. Even then it ignores Doppler effects, and presumes ECG gating so that comparisons are made from the same point in the cardiac cycle.

Reviewing the actual clinical situation in an echo contrast study, it becomes clear that the contrast agent will occupy more than just a small volume. More typically it will fill the entire myocardium or renal parenchyma. Reviewing again Figure 2 note that the incident intensity is diminished proportionally as it passes through each successive small volume. Its magnitude must be described by an exponentially decaying function along the path perfused with contrast agent. A more exact formulation is presented in Figure 5. The path factors unaffected by contrast agent injection are lumped together as 'P-A-F^2' (Path-Attenuation-Factor). Relative intensity can then be expressed simply in terms of bubble concentration N and two constant parameters K_1 and K_2 determined by the distance into the contrast volume, bubble size, fixed path factors, etc.

$$I_R/I_T = NK_1e^{-NK_2}$$

Note that the relative intensity is not simply proportional to N the bubble (and thus contrast agent) concentration. Indeed, above a certain concentration the intensity will actually decrease. This has been observed by the authors in the course of *in vitro* experiments.

18

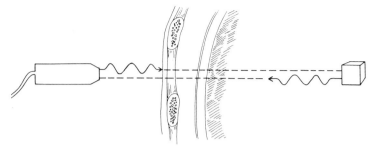

Power-Received = Power-Transmitted x Transmission-Geometry-Fact
x Path-Attenuation-Factor^2
x Volume-Backscatter-Ratio
x Reception-Geometry-Factor

Fig. 4. Schematic depiction of acoustic factors for situation pictured in Figure 3.

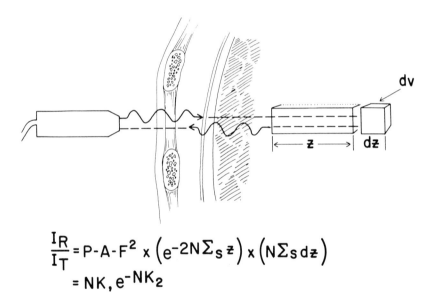

$$\frac{I_R}{I_T}=P\text{-}A\text{-}F^2 \times \left(e^{-2N\Sigma_s z}\right) \times \left(N\Sigma_s dz\right)$$
$$= NK_1 e^{-NK_2}$$

Fig. 5. Relation of received ultrasound intensity (I_r) to transmitted intensity (I_t) as a function of Path Attenuation Factor (P-A-F), microbubble concentration (N), cross-sectional area (Σ_s), and acoustic path through contrast agent.

Experimental setup to test formulas

A bench setup (Figure 6) using an ultrasound transceiver connected to an oscilloscope allowed direct recording of the radiofrequency (rf) signal. A 3.5 MHz transducer was positioned to operate in far-field in a cylinder holding a one-liter solution of 70% Sorbitol. (Sorbitol was chosen because it sustains

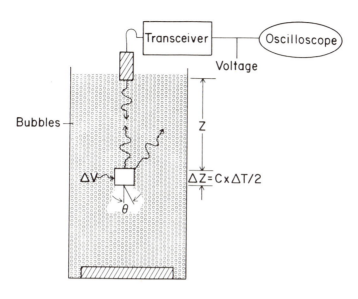

Fig. 6. Schematic depiction of apparatus for measuring reflected ultrasound signal in a beaker of contrast agent.

uniformly small and stable microbubbles.) The Sorbitol was sonicated serially to produce increasing microbubble concentrations. As rf measurements were recorded, simultaneous hemocytometer counts were performed to determine the actual bubble concentration. The rf signal was recorded by taking Polaroid™ pictures of the oscilloscope at constant settings throughout the experiment. These photographs were analyzed by quantitating the largest deflection in the area corresponding to the target volume, and then normalizing so that the largest of all the deflections became 1.0. Each measured deflection is implicitly an average because the camera recorded a number of superimposed tracings.

The graph in Figure 7 shows the results obtained, with normalized rf signal plotted along the vertical axis and bubble concentration plotted along the horizontal axis. The open circles represent the observed data points. The predicted curve is based on the $NK_1e^{-NK_2}$ formula derived above. The data shows a rapid rise in signal, a peak region, and then a region of decreasing signal as concentration increases, as expected from the formula.

The formula also implies that the constants K_1 and K_2 can be determined from the data simply by examining the peak point. In doing so, a good fit is obtained up to a concentration limit. Above that concentration limit, the signal falls off more rapidly than predicted, due to the assumption of single scattering. During the experiment, the Sorbitol actually becomes visibly opaque due to the large number of bubbles, which scattered only a single time. A non-linear least squares fit was done to confirm the peak fit (having eliminated data affected by multiple scattering) resulting in less than a one percent change in the estimation of the peak.

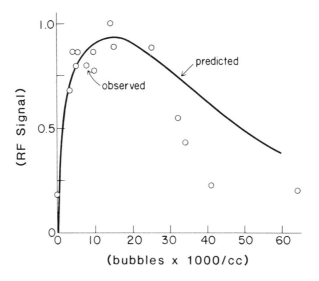

Fig. 7. Plot of radio frequency signal (normalized) versus microbubble concentration.

The next important factor to consider is that the bubbles are randomly arrayed along the ultrasound's path (Figure 8). Thus, instead of just multiplying the Rayleigh scattering formula by concentration times target volume, there is a diminution by factors dependent on the square of the wave number times the bubbles radius [26, 27, and Ishimaru, 28 for treatment of more general problems of random scatters].

The random scattering intensity formulas can be combined with the formula for reflected intensity by integrating the scattered intensity over a large sphere. The

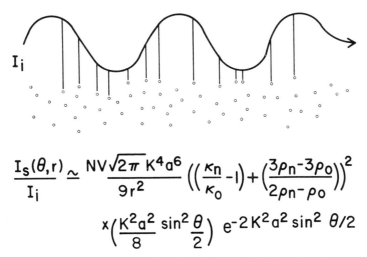

$$\frac{I_s(\theta,r)}{I_i} \sim \frac{NV\sqrt{2\pi}\,K^4a^6}{9r^2}\left(\left(\frac{\kappa_n}{\kappa_0}-1\right)+\left(\frac{3\rho_n-3\rho_0}{2\rho_n-\rho_0}\right)\right)^2$$

$$\times\left(\frac{K^2a^2}{8}\sin^2\frac{\theta}{2}\right)e^{-2K^2a^2\sin^2\theta/2}$$

Fig. 8. Rayleigh scattering by a large number of randomly placed bubbles. Notations are the same as in Figure 1.

resultant cross-section stands in place of the assumed one when the bubbles were treated as little 'mirrors'. When the calculations are carried out, the experimentally observed peak would lead to a prediction of bubble radius that is within a factor of two of the published value, despite the calculation's dependence on not only single scattering, but the more stringent Born Approximation that the incident wave be effectively unaffected by the scattering.

Sonicated microbubble agents

Sonicated microbubble contrast agents can be better appreciated having reviewed contrast agent acoustics. Their obvious advantage over previous agents is their small, red cell sized bubbles which can pass unimpeded through the capillary circulation. The acoustic scattering formulas indicate that reflectance is highly dependent on bubble (or particle) size. This sixth power dependance could easily overshadow sample to sample variation in concentration. Thus there is a distinct benefit to the tighter bubble size distribution in sonicated agents.

The size distributions for some representative sonicated agents are presented in Figure 9; the distribution for a hand-agitated agent is given for comparison [11]. The inherent difficulties in sizing small, highly refractile (in some cases evanescent) bubbles should be recognized in evaluating these reports. Direct observation with a light microscope is the simplest technique (and so recommended as a quick check on agent quality immediately prior to use) but subject to the greatest error. The Coulter Counter™ is perhaps the most widely used instrument for sizing and counting small particles, but its use is confounded by the viscous nature of some of the agents and the effect of the carrier solution on the agents. 'Contaminant' microparticles, present even in intravenous solutions [29], further complicate the use of particle counters. *In situ* laser particle counters [30] have an advantage if the number of bubbles to be counted is kept small. Dilution is not a simple matter with the more viscous agents.

The status of commercially developed agents is not clear; sizes as small as 10 μ have been reported. Data available on transit times are not consistent with unimpeded capillary passage. Whether this is an issue of size, shape, stiffness, or 'stickiness' is unknown.

The sonicated albumin contrast agent reported by Keller et al. [23] is the smallest (4μ ± 2) known bubble/particle agent. It is a more stable reflector and also is smaller than a red cell. The nature of its 'shell' is not understood yet, making detailed acoustic analysis impossible.

In summary, sonicated microbubble contrast agents can be acoustically modeled as a random collection of Rayleigh scatters. Hand-agitated microbubbles have a broader size distribution which complicates the models. Data is not yet available to allow careful acoustic characterization of commercial agents. Those agents with a shell or future agents with layers require a more involved acoustic

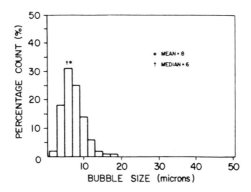

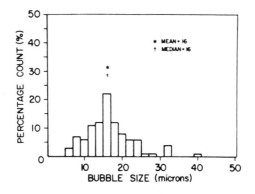

MICROSCOPIC ANALYSIS				
Agent	n	mean°	mode°	persistence
Sorbitol 70% (sonicated)	350	8±2	4	80%
Sorbitol 70% diluted 1:1 with D5W (sonicated)	377	11±7	12	69%
Sorbitol 70% (hand agitated)	211	23±24	12	92%
Dextrose 70% (sonicated)	388	8±3	6	57%
Dextose 50% (sonicated)	198	12±6	8	63%
Renografin-76 (sonicated)	328	10±6	8	58%
Renografin-76 diluted 1:1 with saline	326	13±5	12	42%
Renografin-76 diluted 1:1 with saline (hand agitated)	295	17±13	16	50%

° micron

Fig. 9. Microbubble size distributions.

analysis of the individual bubble/particle's scattering cross section, but can otherwise be modeled like microbubble agents.

Ultrasound imaging system properties

Existing ultrasound systems are inherently volume samplers sensitive to acoustic impedance inhomogeneities. Thus, they are more akin to MRI, CT, and PET scanners than conventional X-ray or gamma-ray scintillation cameras which view a projection. This is significant in that one projection image can (if large enough) capture all the information about all the injected contrast agent at any one instant. A volume sampler can only detect the contrast present in a particular volume at a particular instant and so requires other information (or assumptions) about agent distribution to allow a quantitative analysis.

It is helpful to remember that ultrasound systems detect acoustic energy reflected/scattered by impedance variations (ignoring experimental transmission systems). Current echo contrast agents are effective only to the extent that they suspend acoustic inhomogeneities (gas/solid) in an injectable fluid that flows through the vasculature. There are alternatives. A homogeneous contrast agent would produce an absence of signal as it flowed into a cavity, but could produce a large signal as it flowed through a capillary bed increasing the impedance mismatch between tissue and vascular space.

Current ultrasound scanners have to be adapted to the task of perfusion imaging. They sense the ultrasound energy reflected at impedance inhomogeneities and show varying degrees of brightness in an image that correlates with anatomy. The anatomic accuracy of the image depends on the uniformity of the speed of sound throughout the tissues. The 'accuracy' of the brightness displayed is a purely subjective question. An ultrasound perfusion imaging system, however, must infer contrast agent concentration from the information about induced impedance mismatches. This processing is at least as sophisticated as digital subtraction imaging. It also implies that the signal processing is designed to represent accurately the amount of ultrasonic energy received at the transducer, without consideration to the viewer.

Current scanners introduce two major types of distortion: signal compression and video enhancement. The large dynamic range (about 120dB) of the received signal necessitates some compression to allow processing with available components and also some signal compression to allow human viewing via cathode ray tube. The first type of compression may continue to be necessary, but it must be reversible for calculations. Compression to allow viewing can be eliminated. Video enhancement can also be eliminated. The last is a major impediment to quantitative analysis via commercially available offline processors.

Figure 10 shows the block diagram of a typical ultrasound scanner adapted for perfusion imaging by the addition of a second signal path for quantitative data

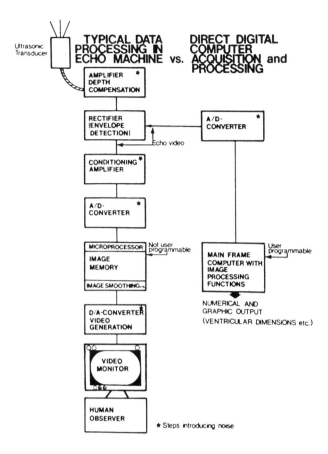

Fig. 10. Computer acquisition of echocardiographic data. Reprinted with permission of author, Dr. A.J. Buda, and publisher [31].

[31]. The original video path remains to allow normal studies and to allow orientation of the transducer during a contrast study. This eliminates any requirement for the perfusion calculations to be done in real time. The only speed requirement is that some partial calculation be rapid enough to allow confirmation of data collection before dismissing the patient. Complete, precise calculation of regional perfusion could be handled by an offline computer.

The major engineering problem is that the quantitative data accumulates very quickly. Signal power information (rectified radio frequency envelope) has to be digitized about three million times per second to resolve one millimeter structures. Commercial scanners can do this and better. Operating at this rate, a commercial scanner will produce about fifty thousand digital samples per sector scan. At thirty scans per second, this gives an overall data rate of one and a half million samples per second. A single sample is between six and twelve bits of information. Assuming an eight bit sample size (256 discrete signal levels), this data rate translates into more than one floppy diskette or twenty-five meters of magnetic tape per second (standard half inch, 1600 bpi). This is actually two to four times faster than readily available floppy disk drives and ten times faster than most tape drives. Multiple head, Winchester disk drives and solid state memory are the usual means of recording data at this rate. Multiple head disks can store very large amounts of data, but are too delicate to move around the hospital. Solid state memory is very fast and can be quite rugged, but is quite expensive in large quantity (e.g., fifty million bytes). Some trade-off is required.

The expected steps required to produce a perfusion image follow. Obtain a baseline image data. For a cardiac exam, capture end-diastolic and/or end-systolic data for a few cycles. Inject a known amount of contrast agent. The volume of dilution must be known for the injection route chosen. Collect image data as the contrast flows in and then washes out of the organ. For cardiac exams, ECG gating to select end-diastolic and/or end-systolic data is likely to be necessary. Display some simple indicator of study quality such as the ratio of signal change with contrast to baseline variation (beat to beat). Depending on the result, further injections can be tried, or the exam may be considered complete. Actual computation of perfusion will first require correction for any distortion inherent in the ultrasound receiver. The effects of time gain compensation (TGC) and signal compression can be reversed at this point.

Some form of rational gain compensation (RGC) can be applied to partially correct for proximal attentuation, so that the difference between contrast images and baseline becomes (to a very simple approximation) directly related to the concentration of microbubbles. This can be used with Fick's principle given the original concentration and the volume of dilution for the injection.

Investigators using digital subtraction angiography have noted the problems of image registration. This is ameliorated somewhat by using a mean baseline image and filtering out fine detail [32].

Unresolved problems

Presuming a suitably chosen contrast agent and a suitably constructed ultrasound scanner some major problems still will require resolution. The foremost problem is how to verify the actual results. Microsphere trapping in the capillary circulation is not quite the same as actual red cell flow [33]. Yet this may be the closest technique for comparison of quantitative perfusion. This will be particularly problematic when trying to investigate variations of flow within a cardiac cycle. Microbubbles presumably flex and follow the red cell flow even during contraction. The other unresolved issue is whether much more involved calculations will be required to decipher contrast images. RGC is really just the first step on the way to estimating acoustic impedance, increment by increment, along the ultrasound path. Computationally this is somewhat simpler than computed to-

26

mography. However, it does not admit to simple closed-form solution as multiple discontinuities are taken into account.

Conclusions

Quantitative ultrasound perfusion imaging is achievable through:
1. Formal acoustic analysis
2. Attention to contrast agent characteristics
3. Attention to equipment transfer function
4. Suitable data acquisition and analysis

References

1. Gramiak R, Shah PM: Echocardiography of the aortic root. Invest Radiol 1968; 3: 356–66.
2. Ziskin MC, Bonakdarpour A, Weinstein DP, Lynch PR: Contrast agents for diagnostic ultrasound. Invest Radiol 1971; 7: 500–5.
3. Meltzer RS, Tickner EG, Sahines TP: The source of ultrasound contrast effect. J Clin Ultrasound 1980; 8: 121–7.
4. Reid CL, Kawanishi DT, McKay CR, Elkayam U, Rahimtoola SH, Chandaratna PAN: Accuracy of evaluation of the presence and severity of aortic and mitral regurgitation by contrast 2-dimensional echocardiography. Am J Cardiol 1983; 52: 519.
5. Kerber RE, Kioschos JM, Lauer RM: Use of an ultrasonic contrast method in the diagnosis of valvular regurgitation and intracardiac shunts. Am J Cardiol 1974; 34: 722–7.
6. Armstrong W, Mueller T, Kinney E, Tickner G, Dillon J, Feigenbaum H: Assessment of myocardial perfusion abnormalities with contrast enhanced two-dimensional echocardiography. Circulation 1982; 66: 166–73.
7. Meltzer RS, Vermeulen HJ, Valk NK, Verdoux PD, Lancee CT, Roelandt J: New echocardiographic contrast agents: Transmission through the lungs and myocardial perfusion imaging. J Cardiovascular Ultrasonography 1982; 1: 277–82.
8. Tei C, Kondo S, Meerbaum S, Ong K, Mauer G, Wood F, Skamaki T, Shimoura K, Corday E, Shah PM: Correlation of myocardial echo contrast disappearance rate ('washout') and severity of experimental coronary stenosis. JACC 1984; 3: 39–46.
9. Kaul S, Pandian NG, Okada RD, Pohost GM, Weyman AE: Contrast echocardiography in acute myocardial ischemia: In vivo determination of total left ventricular 'area of risk'. JACC 1984; 4: 1272–82.
10. Kemper AJ, O'Boyle JE, Cohen CA, Taylor A, Parisi AF: Hydrogen peroxide contrast echocardiography: Quantification in vivo of myocardial risk area during coronary occlusion and of the necrotic area remaining after myocardial reperfusion. Circulation 1984; 70: 309–17.
11. Feinstein SB, Ten Cate FJ, Zwehl W, Ong K, Maurer G, Tei C, Shah PM, Meerbaum S, Corday E: 2D contrast echocardiography. I. In vitro development and quantitative analysis of echo contrast agents. JACC 1984; 3(1): 14–20.
12. Tei C, Sakamaki T, Shah PM, Meerbaum S, Shimoura K, Kondo S, Corday E: Myocardial contrast echocardiography. Circulation 1982; 66: 166–74.
13. Sakamaki T, Tei C, Meerbaum S, Shimoura K, Kondo S, Fishbein M, Y-Rit J, Shah PM, Corday E: Verification of myocardial contrast two-dimensional echocardiographic assessment of perfusion defects in ischemic myocardium. JACC 1984; 3: 34–8.

14. Gillam LJ, Kaul S, Fallon JT, Levine RA, Hedley-White ET, Guerrero JL, Weyman AE: Functional and pathologic effects of multiple echocardiographic contrast injections on the myocardium, brain, and kidney. JACC 1985; 6(3): 687–93.

15. Santoso T, Wiratmo B, Mansyur H, Rahman AM, Panggabean M, Abduraham N: Myocardial perfusion imaging in humans by contrast echocardiography using polygelin colloid solution. JACC 1985; 6(3): 612–20.

16. Goldman ME, Mindich BP: Intraoperative cardioplegia contrast echocardiography for assessing myocardial perfusion during heart surgery. JACC 1984; 4: 1029–34.

17. Mattrey RF, Andre MP: Ultrasonic enhancement of myocardial infarction with perfluorocarbon compounds in dogs. Amer J Cardiology 1984; 54(1): 206–10.

18. Feinstein SB, Ong K, Staniloff H, Fujibayashi Y, Zwehl W, Meerbaum S, Corday E, Shah PM: Myocardial contrast echocardiography: Intracoronary injections and examination of microbubble diameters and intensity decay. Journal of Physiologic Imaging (in press 1986).

19. Frederickson ED, McCoy CE, Powsner S, Lang RM, Goldberg LI, Feinstein SB: Distribution of renal cortical blood flow measured by contrast ultrasonography. Presented at the National Meeting of the American Federation for Clinical Research, May 6, 1985, Washington, D.C. Clin Res 1985; 33: 483A.

20. Feinstein SB, Shah PM, Bing RJ, Meerbaum S, Corday E, Chang BL, Santillan G, Fujibayashi Y: Microbubble dynamics visualized in the intact capillary circulation. JACC 1984; 4(3): 595–600.

21. Feinstein SB, Lang RM, Neumann A, Al-Sadir J, Chua KG, Carroll JD, Keller MW, Powsner SM, Borow KM: Intracoronary contrast echocardiography in humans: Perfusion and anatomic correlates. CIRC 1985; 72(4): III–57.

22. Ten Cate FJ, Feinstein SB, Zwehl W, Meerbaum S, Fishbein M, Shah PM: 2D contrast echocardiography. II. Transpulmonary studies. JACC 1984; 3(1): 21–27.

23. Keller MW, Feinstein SB: Personal communication.

24. Fritzsch Th, Lange L, Zimmerman I: A lung-crossing contrast-agent for echocardiography. Ultrasonoor Bull 1985; Special Issue: 3.

25. Rubissow GJ, MacKay RS: Ultrasonic imaging of in vivo bubbles in decrompression sickness. Ultrasonics 1971; 9: 225–234.

26. Rayleigh JWS: The Theory of Sound (1945), 2nd Edition, Dover Publishers, New York.

27. Morse PM and Ingard KV: Theoretical Acoustics (1968), McGraw-Hill, New York.

28. Ishimaru A: Wave Propagation and Scattering in Random Media, Volumes 1 and 2 (1978), Academic Press, New York.

29. Groves MJ: Particulate contamination in intravenous fluids. I. Nature, origin, and hazard. Pharm J 1973; 210: 185–88.

30. Bierlein J: Particle size analysis of engine oils: A supplement to spectrometric analysis. Technical Report Air Force Materials Laboratory 1979; AFML-TR-79-4215.

31. Buda AJ, Delp EJ, Meyer CR, Jenkins JM, Smith DN, Bookstein FL, Pitt B: Automatic computer processing of digital 2-dimensional echocardiograms. Am J Cardiol 1983; 52: 384–9.

32. Maiser JK, Riederer SJ, Enzmann DR, Brody WR: Some useful concepts of matched filtering in intravenous digital subtraction angiography. Invest Radiol 1984; 19: 424–37.

33. Yoshida S, Akizuki S, Gowski D, Downey JM: Discrepancy between microsphere and diffusible tracer estimates of perfusion to ischemic myocardium. Amer J Physiol 1985; 249 (Heart Circ Physiol 18): H255–H264.

3. Computer Techniques in Contrast Echocardiography

Steven B. FEINSTEIN
University of Chicago, USA

The ultimate goal of contrast echocardiography is to produce a quantifiable, volumetric analysis of myocardial perfusion in patients. Since 1968, when contrast echocardiographic observations were first reported by Gramiak and Shah [1], several innovative and promising techniques using contrast echocardiography have been developed to provide qualitative information on myocardial perfusion [2–4]. However, with recent advances made in interventional cardiology the need to quantitate myocardial blood flow has become critical. The acute and chronic management of patients with ischemic heart disease often depends upon accurate, serial and, quantitative measurements of tissue viability.

Current imaging techniques are limited at quantifying tissue perfusion. Coronary angiography provides useful information regarding coronary artery luminal anatomy, bit is fraught with analysis limitations and ultimately does not provide quantitative functional information with regard to tissue viability [5]. Additionally, coronary angiography and nuclear imaging techniques display data in planar formats without the advantage of real time, tomographic analyses. Newer imaging techniques such as positron emission tomography (PET), computerized axial tomography or nuclear magnetic resonance have not yet proven to be clinically feasible or widely available for routine management of patients with ischemic heart disease [6, 7]. Thus, the clinical paradox remains: blood flow and tissue viability cannot be reliably quantified, yet thrombolytic, angioplasty and surgical revascularization therapies designed to preserve tissue continue to flourish. Clearly, the rational management of patients both in acute and chronic settings will depend upon developing appropriate techniques for measuring and imaging tissue blood flow [7].

The earliest efforts using contrast echo techniques to provide quantitative cardiac output correlations with contrast echocardiography were reported by DeMaria et al. [8]. A photometer placed directly on the video screen was used to measure cardiac output by videointensity. The fractional loss of echo contrast material from the left ventricular cavity was correlated with cardiac output. Valvular regurgitation and intracardiac shunt assessment also were performed using similar techniques [9–13].

J. Roelandt (editor), Digital Techniques in Echocardiography. ISBN 0-89838-861-9.

Subsequently, in an effort to quantitate myocardial perfusion, several investigators performed intracoronary injections of ultrasound-reflective microbubbles in the myocardium of dogs [14–18]. The development of small, stable microbubble contrast agents to track actual blood flow opened up new vistas to the researcher and potentially the clinician, and prompted new efforts designed to quantify the relationship between blood flow and these microbubbles.

While videointensity measurements correlated with contrast loss from the left ventricle when compared to cardiac output, a new, computer-assisted analysis was required in order to assess regional blood flow patterns within the myocardium. Ong et al. initiated computer-assisted video techniques designed to provide regional myocardial 'wash out' or decay functions from experimental intracoronary contrast injection in animals [16].

Experimental studies using intracoronary injections of microbubbles to study myocardial perfusion have been performed using 2-D echocardiography. Cross-sectional tomographic images of the myocardium recorded on videotape were digitized by an off-line analysis. For analysis purposes, Ong et al. developed a Medical Data Systems (MDS) A^2 image processing computer with a Nova 4 CPU, 64K words RAM, a frame buffer, and medium-sized disk adapted from the MDS radionuclide imaging equipment. Based on Ong's system, echo images with element resolution varying from 64×64 to 256×256 could be digitized and stored.

Individual, digitized images (frames) of the left ventricular myocardial cross-section were reviewed to identify endocardial and epicardial borders and subdivided into twelve equiangular segments using the center of gravity as anchoring point. The borders were hand drawn assisted by a simple contour detection algorithm and smoothing technique. The average pixel intensities (standard deviation) for each region of each frame were computed and plotted as a function of time. Figure 1 shows the typical time/intensity curve generated from one of the twelve regions of the two-dimensional cross-sectional echocardiographic image. Note the characteristics of the data represented: the relatively flat baseline, followed by an abrupt and brisk rise in intensity, ultimately a decay or 'wash out' of videointensity.

While several parameters of this typical time/intensity curve deserve attention, the focus has centered upon the decay slope of the graph. This decay slope if fit to a monoexponential function, the corresponding decay half time $(T^{1}/_{2})$ is presumed to indicate the degree of myocardial perfusion; a prolonged $T^{1}/_{2}$ time indicating slow flow and washout, a short $T^{1}/_{2}$ indicating fast myocardial blood flow. Several studies have confirmed the usefulness of the monoexponential fit of intensity decay in correlating blood flow in the heart as well as kidney as determined by epicardial flow meters [14–19].

In this early computerized perfusion analysis method, the salient features include: (1) the echocardiogram is recorded on videotape, (2) the videotape is digitized by an offline system, (3) regions of interest are identified and videoin-

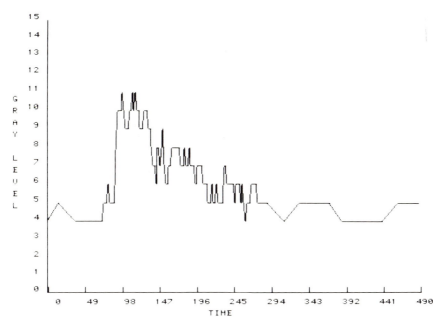

Fig. 1. This time/intensity curve is derived from a digitized 2-D echocardiogram of a myocardial region in a patient with normal coronary anatomy. The baseline intensity is followed by a brisk rise in pixel intensity, signifying the intracoronary injection of sonicated microbubbles. The decay portion follows from the peak and ultimately returns to baseline intensity. The abscicssa is the time in frames (30 frames per second) and the ordinate in pixel intensity using a 16 gray-level display.*

tensity perfusion averages are performed using a semi-automated computer algorithm [20] and (4) a monoexponential function is fit to a portion of the time course of videointensity in the region of interest. Each of these features have a critical effect on the overall analysis and will be reviewed.

The contrast echocardiogram as is currently recorded on videotape is convenient and reliable. No modification of existing ultrasound equipment is required, and 'data' are available for re-analysis. Unfortunately, standards governing the relationship ultrasound signal strength to recorded videointensity do not exist. The various compression, smoothing, and/or edge 'enhancement' circuits used to process the signal before it is finally recorded may entirely distort and compress data. The characteristics of each ultrasound manufacturer dictates the quality of the processed images.

Once the contrast echocardiogram has been recorded on videotape, the study is then digitized for computer analysis. Video frames are recorded at 30 frames a second, each consisting of about a quarter of a million pixels (points). Each of these pixels can take on one of about 250 different intensities (gray-levels), thus occupying about one byte (character) of storage. In other words, one video frame occupies an entire floppy diskette (or a quarter of a new high density diskette)

* The figure is reprinted with permission from the American Journal of Cardiac Imaging 1987; Vol. 1, no. 1, p. 36, fig. 6.

unless a form of data compression is employed. Further, the more time required for myocardial perfusion agents to perfuse the heart, the larger will be the requirements for data storage. By gating the frames of the cardiac cycle, the total amount and speed of data acquisition is significantly reduced. Once the data is acquired, delineating the endo- and epicardial borders to determine intramyocardial perfusion is required. Although several edge detection algorithms exist, border irregularities, noise, and surrounding specular structures make automated edge detection programs time consuming.

The last step in the computer processing of the myocardial enhanced tissue is to determine the change (or lack of change) in videointensity of the myocardium.

Based upon numerous animals intracoronary injections of sonicated microbubbles, the intensity curve is quite consistent in the myocardial tissue [14–16]. Concern for interference by proximal structures and time gain compensation (TGC) distortion leads to the current focus on a time feature rather than simple intensity ratio. Whether intensity rise times corrected for baseline would give a reliable correlate to blood flow is not clear. An empirically applied monoexponential function matched to the major portion of the curve (the decay slope) reduces the noise. From this approach, the investigator has a number of parameters from which to select: (1) time to peak intensity (2) characteristic of the decay portion of the slope (3) selection of appropriate decay function and (4) contingent plans for significant curve irregularities (i.e. intensity drops to baseline prior to curve termination). The choice of the contrast agent, mode of injections and ultrasound artifacts derived from noise or changes in attenuation from proximal structures will to a large extent determine which curve fitting technique is chosen.

Recently, the work in our laboratory at the University of Chicago has employed improved edge detection algorithms [20] and a program for use in an off-line video digitizer system (Franklin Quantic 1200, Bruce Franklin, Inc., Bellevue, WA). The entire injection sequence (20 seconds) is digitized and a series of computer-assisted endocardial and epicardial borders are generated for the entire sequence (maximum 600 frames). The myocardial image is divided into segments by 32 radial cuts and each segment then bisected into a subendocardial and subepicardial region. The average pixel intensity is calculated for the entire sequence for each of the 64 regions. These are processed and displayed as: (1) time/intensity curves for regional myocardial blood flow (dynamic), and (2) cross-sectional myocardial perfusion area (static). After the time/intensity curves are generated, a monoexponential function is fit to the decay slope to obtain a $T^{1/_2}$ (decay rate) using a linear least-squares fit to the logarithm of the curve points.

(1) Regional myocardial blood flow (Dynamic).
Regional blood flow evaluation is based upon individual segment time/intensity curves. Each of the 64 regions shows characteristic pattern consisting of the baseline or pre-injection level, the injection peak, and the ensuing decay portion of the curve. A monoexponential function is applied to the portion of the curve

after the peak and extending to the end of the study. The fit is done by subtracting the pre-injection baseline intensity and then taking the logarithm. A linear, least squarer fit is done to the resultant points. The negative reciprocal of the slope of the least squarer line is proportional to $T^{1/_2}$, the time to decay to one half peak. The $T^{1/_2}$ time is used to assess the relative rate of blood flow within the myocardium. Videotapes of intracoronary injections of sonicated Renografin-76 done during routine coronary catheterization on patients have been analyzed in this manner [2]. Time/intensity curves for each patient from at least two intracoronary injections were obtained. If an intervention is scheduled, such as percutaneous transluminal coronary angioplasty (PTCA) [21] or a pharmacologic approach like an intravascular injection of nitroglycerin, the intracoronary injections are repeated and the time/intensity curves obtained again. $T^{1/_2}$ values are derived from all of the curves and compared to the baseline values for that subject.

(2) Cross-sectional myocardial perfusion area (static).
The analysis program attempts to dramatically reduce the results to be reviewed by producing a 'parametric' image or map of the myocardial perfusion. Instead of a $T^{1/_2}$ calculation for each region, the program is designed to note whether or not the region showed any significant peak and if so, it 'grades' the region based on how long it remained above a certain threshold level. Each region's 'grade' determines its brightness in the parametric image.

Ultimately, the time and intensity of the videodensitometric analysis is represented in a single cross-sectional image. These computer-derived images were taken from a 42 year old patient without evidence for significant coronary disease (Figures 2a and 2b). Note the image (2a) represents the distribution of myocardial blood flow in the right coronary system (2b), and the left coronary artery distribution. Note that there is a small amount of overlap in the perfusion distribution of both arteries.

The clinical studies, at the University of Chicago, have employed these two measures of videodensitometric analysisto correlate perfusion (cross-sectional myocardial tissue) and coronary anatomy. The following explanation and table illustrates the use of these computer-derived analyses in our clinical research efforts [2].

(3) Correlative studies between anatomy and perfusion.
The standard biplane angiographic coronary artery characteristics are compared to the static and dynamic perfusion characteristics from the contrast echo perfusion studies. The following conditions are compared and analyzed: 1) Regional wall abnormalities, 2) Coronary artery occlusions and corresponding 2-D echo perfusion defects (static determination). 3) Coronary artery stenosis and corresponding 2-D echo blood flow (dynamic determination), and 4) Coronary artery stenosis and corresponding 2-D echo blood measurements prior to, and after, mechanical or pharmacologic interventions such as percutaneous transluminal

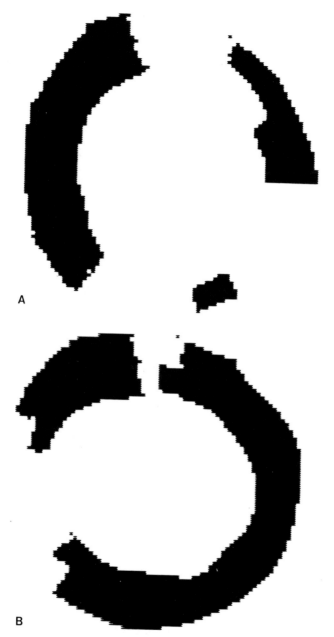

A

B

Fig. 2a. This computer processed cross-sectional myocardial perfusion image is taken from an intracoronary injection of sonicated microbubbles of Renografin-76 in a patient undergoing coronary angiography. The darkened areas represent myocardial perfusion.

Fig. 2b. The right coronary perfusion area is characterized by this computer derived video-intensity mapping. The areas perfused with microbubbles are darkened.

The figure is reprinted with permission from the American Journal of Cardiac Imaging 1987; Vol. 1, no. 1, p. 34, fig. 4 (A) and (B).

coronary angioplasty, or thrombolytic therapy or coronary vasodilator therapy. The following results table describes the comparative studies of anatomy and perfusion:

Table 1. Perfusion/anatomy correlates. Myocardial perfusion and coronary anatomy (from the angiogram) are compared in this manner:

Clinical issue	Coronary angiogram	2-D echo perfusion
1. Overall LV function	Regional wall motion	Regional wall motion & thickness
2. Anatomy/perfusion	Coronary occlusion	Cross-sectional perfusion area (static method)
	Coronary stenosis	Regional myocardial blood flow (dynamic method)

While videodensity measurements continue to provide a semi-quantitative analysis of perfusion based upon the reflectance patterns of echo contrast agents within the myocardium, the ultimate goal of using contrast echocardiography to produce a quantifiable volumetric analysis of myocardial perfusion will require attention to four distinct areas:
1) Production and standardization of quantifiable echo contrast agents
2) Elucidation of the relationship between echo contrast agents and backscatter
3) Establishment of relationship between blood flow and microbubble flow
4) Rectifying the signal processing transformations within the present commercial ultrasound scanners.

Recently, ultrasonic cavitation (sonication) has been applied to liquid solutions in an effort to produce microbubbles which are relatively stable, small and capable of surviving both intracoronary injections and intravenous (or transpulmonary) injections intact. These sonicated microbubbles have proved to be quantifiable echo contrast material (see chapter on the Development of Echo Contrast Agents), and have been used to study myocardial perfusion in the context of varying degrees of coronary artery stenosis [15], valvular regurgitation [22] and renal perfusion [19]. Early studies had documented the ability of these sonicated contrast agents to pass without hindrance through the capillary circulation [23].

A Coulter counter analysis of sonicated albumin is displayed in Figure 3. The albumin microspheres readily pass through the lungs of dogs and subsequently perfuse the myocardial tissue [24]. While these microspheres require further development and investigation before clinical studies can begun, the identification of a prototype agent for future use in contrast echo imaging of left heart structures from an intravenous site is a major step forward in providing a non-invasive quantitation of myocardial perfusion.

The second issue necessary to perform a quantitative analysis is that of estab-

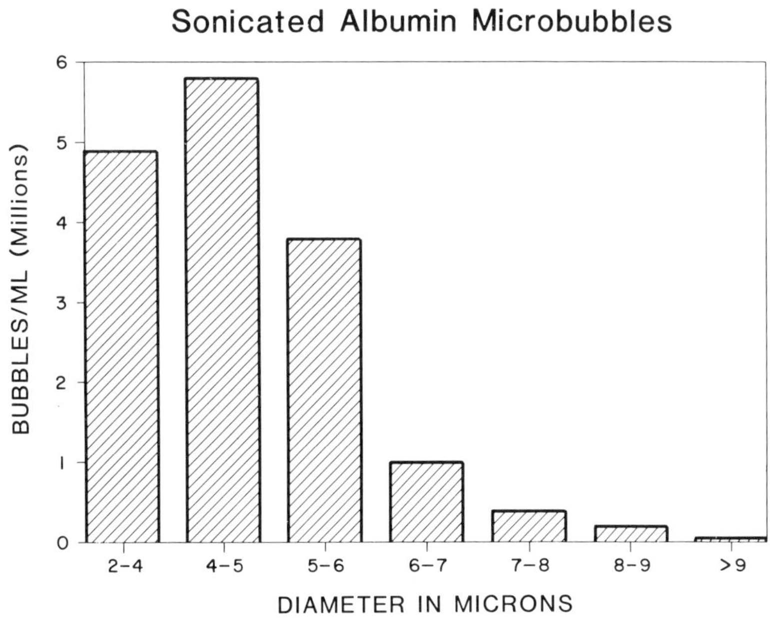

Sonicated Albumin Microbubbles

Fig. 3. A Coulter counter analysis of sonicated microbubbles is displayed as number of bubbles (bubbles/ml) versus diameter (in microns). Few microbubbles were counted above 9 microns in diameter and the majority appear to be between 2 and 6 microns.

lishing the relationship between the microbubbles and the ultrasound backscatter. Based upon the direct, radiofrequency analysis of the absolute size and concentration of microbubbles, a mathematical relationship based on Rayleigh's work [25] could be demonstrated empirically (see also chapter on Quantitation Assessment of Echo Contrast Agents). The mathematical work by Powsner et al. [26] was not feasible until a stable, quantifiable echo contrast agent was developed. Subsequently, the direct radiofrequency backscatter analysis can be applied to tissue structures in order to extend the in vitro research to the clinical theater.

Third, the relationship between the arterial blood flow and the microbubble flow has been demonstrated in two organ structures by correlating electromagnetic flow measurements to videodensity decay [15, 19]. The size and logarithmic half life (or $T^{1}/_2$) of videodensity decay have been correlated in direct intracoronary injections and aortic root injections [14, 27]. From this data, it appears that microbubble size is a critical determinant in establishing physiologic blood flow imaging. When the blood flow was pharmacologically altered in the kidney, a direct relationship was noted between total renal blood flow (by electromagnetic flow) and videodensity decay [19].

Finally, the commercially available ultrasound units display the received data in a compressed, distorted manner that precludes rational data reconstruction from ultrasonic backscatter of echo contrast material within tissue structures. Earlier work by Buda et al. [28] and Miller et al. [29] have recommended direct data acquisition of the ultrasound backscatter energy, prior to pre- and post-processing effects, thus avoiding loss and distortion of data. Several centers and commercial ultrasound companies have identified these issues and are, in fact, moving rapidly to offer both visual as well as 'electronic' images to display data.

These animal results, using direct 'raw' echo signal acquisition have shown promising results in the field of tissue characterization. In addition, the ability to differentiate normally perfused tissue from ischemic tissue is actively being investigated [30]. Although untested, in theory, the use of our ultrasonic tracer substance (i.e., microbubble) may complement the ongoing work in tissue characterization by supplying an intravascular, echogenic tracer substance. The advantage of adding contrast echo to tissue characterization studies may result in a more detailed analysis of the tissue structure and the functional flow compartments.

Ultimately, the progress made to date offers significant promise for the future use of contrast echo techniques to provide a quantifiable, volumetric analysis of myocardial perfusion in man. The advances made in contrast agent preparation and data acquisition and analysis make these research tools, now more clinical applicable. These developments must now keep pace with the clinical use of contrast echocardiography in studying myocardial perfusion in the catheterization laboratory and operation room [2–4].

References

1. Gramiak R, Shah PM: Echocardiography of the aortic root. Invest Radiol 1968; 3: 356–66.
2. Feinstein SB, Lang RM, Neumann A, Al-Sadir J, Chua KG, Carroll JD, Keller MW, Powsner SM, Borow KM: Intracoronary contrast echocardiography in humans: Perfusion and anatomic correlates. Circulation 1985; 72: III–227.
3. Goldman M, Mindich B: Intraoperative cardioplegia contrast echocardiography for assessing myocardial perfusion during heart surgery. JACC 1984; 4: 1029–34.
4. Santoso T, Wiratmo B, Mansyur H, Rahman AM, Panggabean M, Abduraham N: Use of polygelin colloid solution for contrast echocardiographic myocardial perfusion imaging in human. Eur Heart J 1984; 5(1): 1055 (Abstract).
5. White CW, Creighton WB, Doty DB, Hiratza LF, Eastham CL, Harrison DG, Marcks ML: Does visual interpretation of the coronary angiogram predict the physiologic importance of a coronary stenosis? NEJM 1984; 310: 819–24.
6. Skorton DJ, Collins SM: New directions in cardiac imaging. Ann Int Med 1985; 102: 795–9.
7. Laffel GL, Braunwald E: Thrombolytic therapy, a new strategy for the treatment of acute myocardial infarction. NEJM 1984; 311: 770–6.
8. DeMaria AN, Bommer W, Rasor J, Tickner EG, Mason DT: Determination of cardiac output by two-dimensional contrast echocardiography. In Contrast Echocardiography. Meltzer RS, Roelandt J (eds.), The Hague: Martinus Nijhoff, 1982: 289–97.
9. Goldman ME, Mindich BP: Intraoperative contrast echocardiography to evaluate mitral valve operations. JACC 1984; 4: 1035–40.

38

10. Kerber RE, Kioschos JM, Lauer RM: Use of an ultrasonic contrast method in the diagnosis of valvular regurgitation and intracardiac shunts. Am J Cardiol 1974; 34: 722–7.
11. Reid CL, Kawanishi DT, McKay CR, Elkayam U, Rahimtoola SH, Chanraratna PAN: Accuracy of evaluation of the presence and severity of aortic and mitral regurgitation by contrast 2-dimensional echocardiography. Am J Cardiol 1983; 52: 519.
12. Roelandt J: Contrast echocardiography. J Ultrasound in Med and Biol 1982; 3: 1219–26.
13. Sahn DJ, Valdez-Cruz LM: Ultrasonic contrast studies for the detection of cardiac shunts. JACC 1984; 3: 978–85.
14. Feinstein SB, Ong K, Staniloff HM, Fujibayashi Y, Zwehl W, Meerbaum S, Shah PM: Myocardial contrast echocardiography: Examination of intracoronary injections, microbubble diameters, and video-intensity decay. Journal of Physiologic Imaging, 1986 (in press).
15. Ten Cate FJ, Drury JK, Meerbaum S, Noordsy J, Feinstein SB, Shah PM, Corday E: Myocardial contrast two-dimensional echocardiography: Experimental examination at different coronary flow levels. JACC 1984; 60: 418–29.
16. Ong K, Maurer G, Feinstein SB, Zwehl W, Meerbaum S, Corday E: Computer methods for myocardial contrast two-dimensional echocardiography. JACC 1984; 3(5): 1212–18.
17. Maurer G, Ong K, Haendchen R, Torres M, Tei C, Wood F, Meerbaum S, Shah PM, Corday E: Myocardial contrast two-dimensional echocardiography: Comparison of contrast disappearance rates in normal and underperfused myocardium. Circulation 1984; 69: 418–29.
18. Tei C, Sakamaki T, Shah PM, Meerbaum S, Shimour K, Kondo S, Corday E: Myocardial contrast echocardiography. Circulation 1982; 66: 166–74.
19. Frederickson ED, McCoy CE, Powsner SM, Lang RM, Goldberg LI, Feinstein SB: Distribution of renal cortical blood flow, measured by contrast ultrasonography. Clin Res 1984; 33(2): 483A (abstract).
20. Geiser EA, Oliver LH, Gaudin JM, Parisi AF, Reichek N, Weyman AE, Werner JA, Kerber RE, Conti CR: Computer automated endocardial edge defection from 2D echocardiograms: Effective reduction in sequential area and shape variability for wall motion analysis. Clin Res 1984; 32(2): 167A (Abstract).
21. Lang RM, Feinstein SB, Feldman T, Neumann A, Chua KG, Borow KM: Contrast echocardiography for evaluation of myocardial perfusion: Effects of coronary angioplasty. JACC 1986 (in press).
22. Williams KA, Feinstein SB, Neumann A, Carroll JD, Frier PAS, Kremser CB, Al-Sadir J, Chua KG, Borow KM: Microbubble contrast echocardiography for the assessment of valvular regurgitation: Comparison with cineangiography and Doppler echocardiography. Clin Res 1985; 33(2): 238A.
23. Feinstein SB, Shah PM, Bing RJ, Meerbaum S, Corday E, Chang B, Santillan G, Fujibayashi Y: Microbubble dynamics visualized in the intact capillary circulation. JACC 1984; 4: 595–600.
24. Keller MW, Feinstein SB: Successful transpulmonary contrast echocardiography for quantitation of myocardial perfusion. Clin Res 1986 (in press).
25. Rayleigh JWS: The Theory of Sound, 2nd Ed. (1945). Dover, p. 272.
26. Powsner SM, Feinstein SB, Saniie J: Quantitative radiofrequency analysis of sonicated echo contrast agents. JACC 1985; 5: 474 (Abstract).
27. Feinstein SB, Lang RM, Geiser E, Powsner S, Neumann A, Borow KM: A new method for real time of regional myocardial perfusion. JACC 1986; 72(2): Suppl A: 189A.
28. Buda AJ, Delp EJ, Meyer CR, Jenkins JM, Smith DN, Bookstein FL, Pitt B: Automatic computer processing of digital 2-dimensional echocardiograms. Am J Cardiol 1983; 52: 384–9.
29. Miller J, Perez JE, Sobel BE: Ultrasound backscatter of myocardial tissue. Progress in Cardiovascular Disease 1985; 18: 85–110.
30. Rasmussen S, Lovelace DE, Knoebel SB, Ransburg R, Corya BC: Echocardiographic detection of ischemic and infarcted myocardium. JACC 1984; 3(3): 733–43.

4. Myocardial Contrast 2-Dimensional Echocardiography: Analysis of Myocardial Perfusion

Folkert J. TEN CATE
Erasmus University, Rotterdam, The Netherlands

Introduction

Recent interest has evolved to expand the use of 2D-echocardiography (2DE) from measurements of left ventricular (LV) regional and global myocardial function to the study of myocardial perfusion using contrast 2DE [1–5]. Although the first initial reports [6–11] have stimulated great interest to develop a method serving the purpose of measurement of myocardial perfusion, numerous problems since then have arisen. It is the purpose of this report to critically discuss current available litterature and experience in studying myocardial perfusion by contrast 2DE and furthermore evaluate current and future research opportunities to develop an echocontrast method for measuring myocardial perfusion.

Myocardial contrast 2DE (MC-2DE)

After the first report of de Maria and Bommer [6] who injected echocontrast into the myocardium and observed subsequent myocardial contrast enhancement a number of authors have described myocardial contrast 2DE studies using various contrast agents, various ways of injections and various methods of analysis [6–11]. In this way the results of these studies can hardly be compared to each other. This urges the development of a standardized route of injection using standard echocontrastagents with known microbubble size and quantity. Moreover most authors have studied MC-2DE using fixed coronary artery stenosis [7–10] or measuring infarct size [12], whereas only one experimental study is available [10] where MC-2DE have been studied at various levels of epicardial coronary flow.

Route of injection

De Maria and Bommer [6] measured myocardial contrast effect after intracardiac or intracoronary injections; Armstrong [7] used aortic root injections whereas

J. Roelandt (editor), Digital Techniques in Echocardiography. ISBN 0-89838-861-9.

Maurer, Tei and Ten Cate all reporting from the same laboratory [8–10] used intracoronary injections although the echocontrast agent used differed. A measurable although not analyzable myocardial contrast effect has been obtained after intravenous injections [13] and after injections into a peripheral pulmonary artery branch [14].

Method of analysis

Bommer and Armstrong [6, 7] analyzed their images by manually manipulating an analog videodensitometer over the videoscreen, whereas others [8–10] used a digitized computerized 2DE contrast method including digital subtraction of videodensity images as developed by Ong [15]. These last three authors took advantage of this method to quantify the appearance and disappearance of the contrast effect by a method similar to the analysis of indicator dilutioncurves [10]. The limitations of this method have been described and presented [10].

Reported values for normal and underperfused myocardium

Armstrong [7] found a correlation between measured lightintensity and myocardial blood flow as measured by radioactive microspheres and he indicated that areas of decreased blood flow showed also decreased videodensity. Most authors [8–10] showed significant delay of contrast disappearance in underperfused myocardium as compared to normally perfused myocardium (see Table 1 and 2). Hyperemia shortened myocardial contrast disappearance time [10] but it did not change its value when compared to normal perfusion [16] in a recent study.

Using the same experimental preparation and method of analysis values for

Table 1. Myocardial contrast studies.

A.	Experimental data	Myocardial enhancement	I/S/H
	de Maria and Bommer	+	I/S
	Meltzer	+	not mentioned
	Armstrong	+	S/I
	Tei	+	S/I
	Maurer	+	S/I
	Ten Cate	+	S/I/H
	Schartl	+	H
B.	Human data		
	Matsumoto	+	I
	Santoso	+	–

I = Ischemia; S = fixed coronary stenosis; H = Hyperemia. For details see text.

normal myocardial perfusion (indicated as T1/2, decay rate calculated from the myocardial contrast appearance and disappearance curve) varied from 22.3 ± 7.0 seconds [9] and 23 ± 6 seconds [17] to 5.2 ± 0.3 seconds [10]. The reported values for T1/2 in underperfused myocardium even varied more. These different values can mainly be attributed to the different echocontrast agents used. Both Maurer [9] and Tei [8, 17] used handagitated renografin/saline solutions (different mixtures of 1 ÷ 1 and 3 ÷ 2 respectively), whereas Ten Cate [10] used a relatively new contrast agent: sonicated Dextrose 50%. Although T1/2 using this newer contrast agent was shorter than in earlier reported studies [8, 9], it was not comparable to transit time of myocardium as measured from radioactive labelled erythrocytes [18], or measured from heat loss and temperature distribution [19]. The reported values for these methods varied from 0.8 to 1.8 seconds.

Regarding the discrepancy between these observations it seems highly premature to study myocardial contrast effect in human beings [20, 21]. Microbubble size of the echocontrast agent used was too large (>30 u) and might obstruct capillary flow and thus disturbs the measurements of the contrast disappearance rate.

Examples of myocardial contrast perfusion studies

For the analysis of myocardial contrast enhancement enddiastolic myocardial images of the shortaxis of the left ventricle were digitized into the echographic computersystem from a point before echocontrast injection until echocontrast has disappeared completely. The echo intensity was measured as mean pixel brightness for each of 12 equal myocardial segments and thereafter segment to segment brightness was plotted for each individual enddiastolic image. This procedure could be repeated at different levels of epicardial coronary artery flow, but for the sake of clarity only the images out of the control flow situations will be described.

T1/2 was calculated from the construction of the time intensity curve (Figure 1)

Table 2. Myocardial echocontrast washout times (T1/2).

	Normal perfusion	Ischemia	Hyperemia
Armstrong	–	–	–
Tei	23 ± 7 s	prolonged	–
Maurer	idem	prolonged	–
Ten Cate	5.2 ± 0.3 s	prolonged	shortened
Schartl	6.5 ± 1.5 s	not mentioned	7.8 ± 0.9 s
Matsumoto	11.0 ± 3.8 s	prolonged	–

s = seconds; T1/2 = halflife of contrast echo disappearance time. For details see text.

42

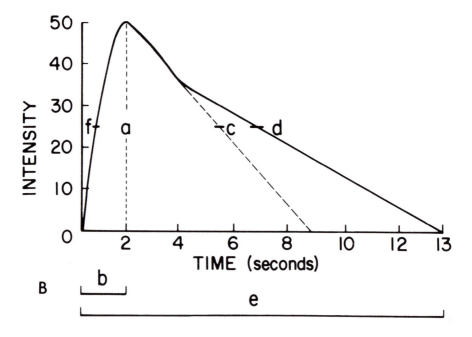

Fig. 1. Schematic drawing of echocontrast time activity curve, indicating that several parts of the curve might be useful for characterization of myocardial blood flow. a = peak intensity; b = time of echocontrast appearance to peak intensity (seconds); c = half life of rapid decay phase (seconds); d = half life of overall decay phase (seconds); e = total duration of echocontrast time activity curve (seconds); f = half life of curve upstroke (seconds). Reproduced with permission from J. Am. Coll. Cardiol. 1984; 3: 1219.

as $T1/2 = \ln 2/k$ where $\ln$ = natural logarithm and k = exponential decay rate [9], using a monoexponential least square fit [15].

From the curve, peak intensity, time from appearance of echocontrast to peak intensity, total curve duration and upstroke half life could be calculated [10]. From our own experience most curves had two components during its decay phase, $T1/2$ was calculated for the first initial fast portion of the curves (Fig. 1). Regarding the many limitations of this method [10, 15] it still was possible to distinct between control coronary flow, ischemia (>50% flow reductions) and hyperemia induced by dipyridamole (>50% flow increase) by calculation of $T1/2$.

The relation between an increased $T1/2$ value and decreased coronary flow and the decreased $T1/2$ with increased coronary flow is nicely illustrated in Figure 2. Not only $T1/2$ but also time to peak contrast effect and overall curve duration were different and also could distinguish between these three flow states. In contrast to Armstrong [7] no distinction could be made between ischemia and normal flow if peak brightness was measured.

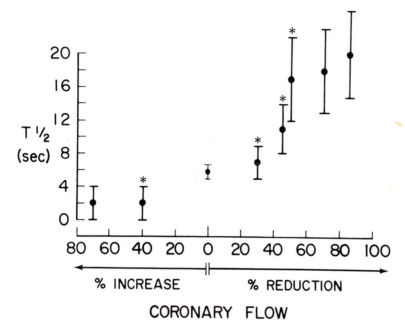

Fig. 2. Relation between percent of coronary flow reduction or increase from the control level and T1/2 for the center of the ischemic zone. Coronary artery flow reduction results in a district increase in T1/2, whereas T1/2 significantly decreases during dypiridamole induced hyperemia. Values are mean ± standard deviation. *p<0.05 compared with control. Reproduced with permission from J. Am. Coll. Cardiol. 1984; 3: 1219.

Echocontrast agent

The ideal echocontrast agent for 2DE myocardial perfusion studies should give quantifiable echocontrast effect (independent of the method of analysis), should not partially or totally obstruct capillary flow, do not give a hyperemic response after injection and should be nontoxic.

Although these qualifications seems logic to understand, at this time no such echocontrast agent exists.

Regarding sizes of 6–8 μ in both canine and human capillaries, the echocontrast agent should contain microbubbles of this size or smaller, to prevent obstruction of capillary flow which potentially invalidates myocardial perfusion studies [22]. Bommer used saccharine encapsulated microballoons of 30 μ, Armstrong gelatinencapsulated balloons of 75 μ, Maurer and Tei microbubbles of 18 to 40 μ and Ten Cate microbubbles of 12 ± 6 μ. The variation of sizes of these microbubbles explains the different 'washout' times published in different studies (Table 2).

Although recently [16] sugar encapsulated microbubbles of small sizes (3 μ) have been used for myocardial perfusion studies the calculated washout times of myocardial contrast were not different between normally and hyperemic myocar-

44

dium. Fluorocarbon particles have been used for myocardial enhancement but the data from this agent are too scarce to draw any conclusions yet.

With better understanding of microbubble physics and the use of highfrequency echotransducers [23] it is expected that in the future also collagen particles, fat emulsions or other solid particles can be used for myocardial perfusion studies.

Assessment of myocardial infarction by myocardial contrast 2DE

After the first initial observations that myocardial perfusion defects could be visualized by contrast 2DE, several authors [12, 24, 25] have reported that myocardial infarctions could be measured by this method with rather good accuracy.

Sakamaki [12] described comparison of myocardial infarct size measured by TTC in pathologic ventricular slabs and equivalent measurements of contrast studies of myocardium. The so called negative contrast area correlated well with the area measured from the pathologic specimen.

The extent of necrosis was slightly overestimated by contrast 2DE. The contrastagent used in this study was hand agitated renografin/saline.

Armstrong [24] reported the same findings using Hydrogen peroxide. He found that the area of infarction measured from the pathologic specimen correlated well with the size of the infarcted area measured from myocardial contrast-2DE, with excellent inter- and intraobserver correlations. Moreover the extent of absent systolic wall thickening correlated well with the extent of infarction, which has been reported earlier in studies not using contrast 2DE.

Kemper [25] using hydrogen peroxide as well found good correlations between echocardiographically determined infarction size and postmorteminfarction size using TTC colouring whereas wallmotion abnormalities were found in under- and nonperfused areas.

Summary and conclusions

Myocardial contrast 2DE seems a useful and promising method to determine myocardial perfusion, in the experimental setting. Until now however, a good, nontoxic reproducible echocontrastagent has not been developed. Future research must focus on the development of these agents.

The figures shown in this article have been obtained during the author's sabattical leave from the Thoraxcenter at Cedars Sinai Medical Center, Los Angeles, Ca., USA.

References

1. Carr K, Engler R, Forsythe J, et al.: Measurements of left ventricular ejection fraction by mechanical cross-sectional echocardiography. Circulation 1979; 59: 1196.
2. Schiller N, Acquatella H, Ports T, et al.: Left ventricular volume from paired biplane two-dimensional echocardiography. Circulation 1979; 60: 547.
3. Gueret P, Meerbaum S, Wyatt HL, et al.: Two-dimensional echocardiographic quantitation of left ventricular volumes and ejection fraction: importance for accounting for dyssupernergy in short axis reconstruction models.
4. Moynihan P. Parisi A, Feldman C: Quantitative detection of regional left ventricular contraction abnormalities by two-dimensional echocardiography. Circulation 1981; 63: 752.
5. Haendchen RV, Wyatt HL, Maurer G, et al.: Quantitation of regional cardiac function by two-dimensional echocardiography. I. Patterns of contraction in the normal left ventricle. Circulation 1983; 67: 1234.
6. De Maria AN, Bommer WJ: Echocardiographic visualization of myocardial perfusion by left heart and intracoronary injections of echocontrast agents. Circulation 1980; 60: III–143 (abstract).
7. Armstrong WF, Mueller TM, Kinney EL, et al.: Assessment of myocardial perfusion abnormalities with contrast-enhanced two-dimensional echocardiography. Circulation 1982; 66: 166.
8. Tei C, Sakamaki T, Shah PM, et al.: A reproducible technique of myocardial opacification for identifying regional perfusion deficits. Circulation 1983; 67: 585.
9. Maurer G, Ong K, Haendchen R, et al.: Myocardial contrast two-dimensional echocardiography: comparison of contrast disappearance rates in normal and underperfused myocardium. Circulation 1984; 69: 418.
10. Ten Cate FJ, Drury K, Meerbaum S, et al.: Myocardial contrast two-dimensional echocardiography: experimental examination at different flow levels. J Am Coll Cardiol 1984; 3: 1219.
11. Meltzer RS, Vermeulen HJ, Valk N, et al.: New echocardiographic contrast agents: transmission through the lung and myocardial perfusion imaging. J Cardiovasc ultrasonography 1982; 1: 277.
12. Sakamaki T, Tei C, Shah PM, et al.: Verification of myocardial contrast two-dimensional echocardiographic assessment of perfusion defects in ischemic myocardium. J Am Coll Cardiol 1984; 3: 34.
13. Valdes Cruz LM, Sahn DJ: Ultrasonic contrast studies for the detection of cardiac shunts. J Am Coll Cardiol 1984; 3: 978.
14. Ten Cate FJ, Feinstein S, Zwehl W, et al.: Two-dimensional echocardiography. II. Transpulmonary studies. J Am Coll Cardiol 1984; 3: 21.
15. Ong K, Maurer G, Feinstein S: Computer methods for myocardial contrast two-dimensional echocardiography. J Am Coll Cardiol 1984; 3: 1212.
16. Schartl M, Miszalok V, Heidelmeier Ch: Quantitative Beurteilung der Myokardperfusion mittels Kontrastechokardiographie. In: Proc. German Heart Assn., 1985.
17. Tei, Kondo S, Meerbaum S, et al.: Correlation of myocardial echocontrast disappearance rate ('wash out') and severity of experimental coronary stenosis. J Amer Coll Cardiol 1984; 3: 39.
18. Sarelius IH, Duling BR: Direct measurement of microvessel hematocrit red cell flux, velocity and transit time. Am J Physiol 1982; 243: H1018.
19. Ten Velden GHM, Elzinga G, Westerhof N: Left ventricular energetics. Heat loss and temperature distribution of canine myocardium. Circ Res 1982; 50: 63.
20. Santoso I, Wiratmo B, Mansyur H, et al.: Use of polygelin colloid solution for contrast echocardiographic myocardial perfusion imaging in human. Eur Heart J 1984; 5 (suppl. I): 196.
21. Matsumoto M, Yasui K, Shimazu T, et al.: Evaluation of severity of coronary stenosis by contrast echomyocardiography in clinical cases. Circulation 1984; 70 (suppl. II): 393.
22. Feinstein SB, Shah PM, Bing RJ, et al.: Microbubble dynamics visualized in the intact capillary circulation. J Amer Coll Cardiol 1984; 4: 595.

46

23. Zwehl W, Areeda J, Schwartz G, et al.: Physical factors influencing quantitation of two-dimensional contrast echo amplitudes. J Amer Coll Cardiol 1984; 4: 157.

24. Armstrong WF, West SR, Dillon JC, et al.: Assessment of location and size of myocardial infarction with contrast-enhanced echocardiography. II. Application of digital imaging techniques. J Amer Coll Cardiol 1984: 4: 141.

25. Kemper AJ, O'Boyle JE, Sharma S, et al.: Hydrogen peroxide contrast enhanced two-dimensional echocardiography: real-time in vivo delineation of regional myocardial perfusion. Circulation 1983; 3: 34.

5. Quantitative Contrast Echocardiography: What can the Practicing Cardiologist expect?

Richard S. MELTZER
Sinai Medical Center, New York, USA

What is quantitative contrast echocardiography?

The contrast echocardiographic effect was first noted by Joyner and first reported by Gramiak and Shah in 1968 [1]. Initially it was used in a largely qualitative manner to answer clinical questions about structure identification, intracardiac shunts, valvular regurgitation, and complex congenital heart disease. These topics have been extensively reviewed [2–6] and will not be covered in this chapter. Suffice it to point out that these initial contrast uses involved answering 'yes-no' questions: 'Does an ASD exist?', 'Is this structure the left main coronary artery?', 'Does this baby have a PDA', etc.

Quantitative contrast echocardiography, as the name implies, involves making measurements from contrast echocardiograms. A great deal more physiologic information is potentially contained in contrast echocardiograms if the cardiologist does not limit analysis to yes-no qualitative questions [7]. Different types of quantitative information can be obtained from M-mode and two-dimensional echocardiograms, which will be separately treated below. Of course, the standard type of time, distance, and slope (velocity) measurements that are used in M-mode echocardiography are used to quantify M-mode contrast effects. Two-dimensional echocardiography has introduced a new quantitative potential that is just beginning to be realized: videodensitometry. Most quantitative contrast echocardiography from two-dimensional echocardiography will be via videodensitometry. The microprocessor technology of newer echocardiographic equipment offers exciting possibilities that researchers are just beginning to work on: at present, most equipment being marketed has the hardware capability to do videodensitometry. In order for videodensitometry to become a clinically useful tool, however, new contrast agents and reproducible techniques of contrast echocardiography must be developed, and the complex relationship between the

This work was partly supported by a Clinician-Scientist Award and Grant-in-Aid 82–1048 from the American Heart Association, by a grant from the Heart Research Foundation, New York, NY, and by an Established Fellowship and Grant-in-Aid from the New York Heart Association.

J. Roelandt (editor), Digital Techniques in Echocardiography. ISBN 0-89838-861-9.

microbubble contrast targets and ultimate videodensity need better definition. If these relationships as well as the microbubble dynamics in the circulation are adequately understood, many of the quantitative contrast echocardiographic applications mentioned in the section on two-dimensional echocardiography will be merely software modifications that might even be retro-fitted to many currently existing echocardiographic systems.

Quantitative M-mode contrast echocardiography

Due to its format, M-mode echocardiography is particularly suited to timing, depth and slope (= velocity) measurements. Specifically, M-mode echo has a much better time resolution (about 1 msec) than 2D echo (about 33 msec). Different types of measurements can be made which reflect different underlying physiologic events. Sections on each of the following measurements that can be made from M-mode echocardiography follow: 1) timing of onset of contrast appearance – with respect to the cardiac cycle; 2) timing of onset of contrast appearance – with respect to different cardiac chambers; 3) relative intensity of contrast specification; 4) clearance time; and 5) velocity from M-mode contrast trajectory slopes.

Timing of onset of contrast appearance with respect to the cardiac cycle

Contrast often appears abruptly on the echocardiogram. It may reproducibly appear during a specific portion of the cardiac cycle even though it was injected peripherally at various times (and not coordinated) with respect to the cardiac cycle. This phenomenon is used to diagnose tricuspid regurgitation (TR) – in patients with TR contrast appears in the IVC at the onset of the 'v' pulsation after peripheral venous injection in the upper extremity [8–10].

Usually ASD's can be distinguished from VSD's on clinical grounds and/or on the basis of the baseline (pre-contrast) echocardiogram. In addition, there are some subtle differences of the timing of the contrast appearance with respect to the cardiac cycle after injections. In an ASD, contrast enters the LV in diastole, after the mitral valve opens. In a VSD the contrast usually appears earlier, during the isovolumic relaxation phase before mitral opening [11]. Serwer et al [12] have even proposed using the timing of appearance of LV contrast after IV injection as a means for estimating the hemodynamics in patients with VSD's usually/there is little or no shunting in patients with RV pressures <60% of LV pressures. Those with RV pressure between 60%–80% of LV pressures (and a pulmonary/septemic flow ratio about 2.0–5.0) had appearance of contrast in the LV during isovolumic relaxation as mentioned above, but the contrast returned to the right heart (was 'cleared') during mid to late diastole, and thus none remained at end-diastole to be ejected into the aorta on the subsequent systole. A third pattern was found in patients with systemic pulmonary pressures and Qp/Qs >3:1 – initial appearance of contrast in the LV during isovolumic relaxation as above, but the contract was not 'cleared' back to the right side during diastole and remained to be ejected into the aorta. A fourth pattern was seen in these with systemic RV pressures and right-to-left shunting (Qp/Qs 0.4–0.8): entry into the LV was seen earlier than in the second or third group. Even earlier entry (with respect to the QRS complex on the ECG) was seen in 34 patients with advanced Eisenmenger syndrome and pulmonary vascular resistance > 15 U/m2. Thus, timing of contrast shunting with respect to the cardiac cycle may help provide information about hemodynamics.

Timing of onset of contrast appearance with respect to different cardiac chambers

In a patient with an ASD, following peripheral IV injection, contrast enters the left heart within the first few cardiac cycles after its appearance in the right heart. Characteristically this delay is longer in patients with pulmonary arteriovenous fistulae [13]. Thus, there is an overlap with a relative delay of 3–5 cardiac cycles where either intercardiac or intrapulmonary shunting may be occurring: clinical correlation and other echocardiographic clues are necessary to differentiate.

Relative intensity of contrast opacification

A cardiac chamber or great vessel often opacify much more or less than another opacified chamber or vessel. This may serve as a marker for the underlying physiology. For example in patients with transposition of the great arteries (TGA), the adequacy of atrial mixing can be judged by assessing the relative intensity of contrast in the aorta and pulmonary artery after peripheral IV contrast injection. Why is this? Because the great vessel with the most intense contrast obviously is receiving most of the systemic venous return, and this is the aorta in patients with uncomplicated TGA. In these ductus-dependent babies without intracardiac shunting, balloon atrial septostomy (Rashkind Procedure) allows mixing at the atrial level. After a successful Rashkind procedure the aorta and pulmonary artery will be opacified to fairly similar intensity [14].

Clearance time

Clearance time may be defined as the length of time or number of cardiac cycles necessary for contrast to be cleared from a vessel or cardiac chamber after its initial appearance. This definition may be difficult to apply in practice, since the end point is poorly defined: contrast usually decays exponentially after its delivery is completed, and exactly where to consider the end is often problematic. We use 2 approaches to aid us here: 1) use the last cardiac cycle where an arbitrary number – perhaps 5 – definite contrast images are seen and call that the end point, or 2) avoid the problem by making observations such as: 'contrast remained for >15 cardiac cycles' or 'all normals cleared contrast in <10 cardiac cycles'.

Both low clearance time and regurgitation of a valve immediately proximal or distal to the chamber or vessel of interest would be expected to prolong the clearance time of contrast from that chamber. For example, IVC and right heart clearance of contrast is prolonged in patients with tricuspid regurgitation, and right ventricular contrast clearance time is also prolonged in right heart failure [15].

The relative clearance time of 2 cardiac chambers or vessels can also be examined. For example, in babies with TGA and minimal interatrial mixing, where the aortic saturation is <40%, the aortic contrast clearance time after IV injection is more than twice the pulmonary contrast clearance time (as mentioned above, the aortic contrast intensity is also greater). When there is more interatrial mixing and aortic oxygen saturation is 40–60%, the pulmonary artery clearance time is more than half that of the aorta. Finally, when mixing is adequate and aortic saturation >60%, both great arteries have similar contrast clearance times (and similar contrast intensities).

Velocity from contrast trajectory slope on M-mode echocardiograms: 'Poor Man's Doppler'

The slope of a contrast trajectory, as an M-mode tracing is the component of the velocity of the microbubble 'service' or contrast projected along the ultrasound beam. Both qualitative information (whether the microbubble is moving toward of away from the transducer) [16, 17] and quantitative information (velocity) [18, 19] can be obtained from this slope analysis. Since the same ultrasound beam can be analyzed to give both M-mode and Doppler information, this provides a simple method for Doppler calibration: slopes of injected contrast can be measured and compared with the Doppler output to see if the velocity measurements are similar.

Quantitative two-dimensional contrast echocardiography

If there were a one-to-one relationship between microbubble concentration and contrast intensity as measured by videodensitometry, then indicator-dilution theory and techniques would be applicable to contrast two-dimensional echocardiography. Unfortunately, this is not the case. The problem is complicated both because microbubbles are not an ideal indicator and because there are many known limitations on videodensitometry as a technique to quantify microbubble concentration. Microbubbles may not distribute uniformly in a blood vessel or cardiac chamber – they have a tendency to rise and larger bubbles rise faster than smaller ones, and at least some bubbles 'marginate' along vein walls after injection, accounting for the familiar clinical observation of increased cardiac contrast density after patient motion, cough, or arm elevation and vein 'milking'. The largest problem is that microbubbles are not inert indicators but have a dynamic equilibrium with the liquid phase around them and grow or decay due to multiple hydrodynamic and physical chemical forces that are incompletely characterized. Sad to say, the current 'state of the art' clinically is that we have minimal control over the size and uniformity of the microbubbles that we inject into patients, and no way to analyze the microbubble size and concentration spectrum either at the point of injection or, more importantly, in the heart when the microbubbles are being imaged. For quantitative contrast echocardiography to become a clinical tool, microbubble monitors will have to be developed at least for in vitro use, and preferably for in vivo applications as well. This is not a trivial task, since existing microbubble monitors using optical, ultrasonic, or laser technology are not suited for contrast echocardiographic applications and dedicated monitors capable of measuring the required microbubble size spectra and concentrations are quite complicated to build, calibrate, and use. Nevertheless, this is a key requirement as a basis for quantitative contrast two-dimensional echocardiography, and is being worked upon in our laboratory and several others.

Once better microbubble monitors exist, the design and study of contrast agents will be significantly aided. Currently there are several approaches to designing new contrast agents: 1) hand agitation and syringe agitation are used clinically but suffer from reproducibility problems, 2) high intensity insonification of liquids creates microbubble suspensions [20], 3) a polysaccharide agent associated with microbubbles when injected intravenously [21], and 4) a precision microbubble generator in which gas is introduced into a flowing liquid stream [22]. Factors such as viscosity, temperature, surface tension, etc. that affect bubble generation for contrast agents are just being looked at in initial studies [23]. A great deal of work needs to be done before we can reliably create contrast agents with a known size and concentration of microbubbles that have a known and reproducible behavior in the bloodstream so that a known size and number of microbubbles can be imaged in the heart.

Even if this formidable task can be overcome, there are significant limitations in ultrasonic imaging and videodensitometric analysis. One obvious extreme is the 'overload' phenomenon recognized by most clinical echocardiographers. This is actually a combination of several different phenomena: 1) At a high microbubble concentration, so much of the ultrasonic energy is reflected that there is insufficient energy left in the beam to image distal structures, 2) Sound travels more slowly through a combined microbubble-blood medium (otherwise stated –

there are multiple internal reflections/refractions and thus a longer sound trajectory) and thus contrast is occasionally displayed artifactually more distal than it is anatomically, 3) the videodisplay cannot display the full dynamic range of returning signals, and thus in clinical ultrasonic images a maximum 'white' is frequently exceeded for all concentrations of microbubbles above the threshold of maximum whiteness that the machine is set to, 4) Amplifier circuitry may be saturated by high-intensity signals introducing distortion even before videodisplay.

Not only the obvious 'overload' limitation must be understood and overcome, but also many more subtle aspects of ultrasonic imaging, beam characteristics and focusing, signal processing in the particular instrument and transducer being used, the effects of intervening structures (chest wall, etc.), preprocessing, postprocessing, gain curves, methods of videodensitometric assignment to each pixel, etc. [24, 25].

Myocardial perfusion imaging

Certainly the most exciting potential application of quantitative contrast echocardiography for the practicing cardiologist is the quantification of myocardial blood flow. Qualitatively, it has been shown that injections in the aortic root or coronary arteries can be imaged as a myocardial contrast blush in experimental animals [26–28] and humans [29, 30]. Various authors have looked quantitatively in experimental animals at the spatial extent of the contrast effect, its videodensitometric intensity, or its kinetics ('washout') to quantify different aspects of myocardial blood flow, coronary blood flow, coronary stenosis, etc. [27, 31–34]. This initial work is quite promising, since before contrast echocardiography it was impossible to even qualitatively evaluate myocardial perfusion abnormalities in real time, and certainly not with relatively inexpensive equipment available already to most cardiologists with excellent temporal and spatial resolution (2D echo instruments).

Where are we going from here in quantitative two-dimensional contrast echocardiography of myocardial perfusion? Probably several directions are important at present. Safety must remain a prime concern. Though it is known that peripheral (intravenous) contrast echocardiography is safe [35], there is little information available about the safety of intracoronary contrast echocardiography. Initial information suggests lack of gross toxicity in humans [29, 30] and animals [36], but other careful animal studies recently reported in preliminary form suggest possible myocardial depression due to echo contrast agents [37, 38]. Careful toxicity studies and methods to prevent coronary air embolus are necessary if myocardial perfusion imaging by contrast echocardiography is to enter clinical use. Probably the initial utility of this invasive technique (intracoronary or aortic root injections) will be in the 'on-line' assessment of myocardial reperfusion during angioplasty or intracoronary thrombolytic therapy. Its initial utility may be both qualitative and quantitative.

An ultimate goal of quantitative contrast echocardiography is this area would be the ability to quantify myocardial blood flow after intravenous injections of agents that pass the pulmonary capillaries and yield a myocardial contrast blush. If this can be done, it would have an obvious major impact on the diagnosis and therapy of coronary disease. Though this goal seems achievable at present, the difficulties and limitations listed in the previous section (as well as others) suggest that years of research remain before this important goal is attained.

Shunt quantification

In one of the initial quantitative two-dimensional contrast echocardiographic studies in 1978, Hagler et al. from the Mayo clinic reported that the magnitude of a left-to-right shunt in 12 patients determined by Fick and indicator-dilution techniques at catheterization correlated well with videodensitometric estimates obtained by analyzing videotaped echo studies obtained during the catheterization [39, 40]. A commercially available videodensitometer was used and the percentage of left-to-right shunt after left heart injection was estimated by dividing the area under the right heart videodensity curve by that under the left heart curve and multiplying by 100. Correlations of r = 0.93 with dye curves (N = 8) and r = 0.91 with Fick estimates (N = 12) were obtained.

In a quantitative M-mode contrast echocardiographic study, Serwer et al. noted a correlation between the timing and persistence of left ventricular contrast after IV injection and the relative right ventricular pressure elevation in ventricular septal defects [41, 42]. Though this is not a direct quantification of the shunt magnitude, it is an important piece of data from quantitative contrast echocardiography important for the practicing cardiologists managing patients with VSDs.

In a more recent quantitative contrast study, Valdes-Cruz and Sahn noted a trend towards a correlation between the pulmonary to systemic flow ratio in a variable size VSD surgically created in 4 dogs and a measure of negative jet size in the RV times a change in videodensity due to the left-to-right shunt [43].

Though these studies suggest that quantitative contrast echocardiography may be useful for some aspects of shunt quantification in the future, several problems need to be overcome if this is to enter clinical practice. The 3 most important are: 1) improving the reliability and reproducibility and bolus injection characteristics (?use of external jugular site) of peripheral contrast injections, 2) attaining transpulmonary transmission of contrast after IV injection to allow quantification of left-to-right shunts, and 3) better definition of the limitations and development of techniques for the use of videodensitometric curves as indicator-dilution curves (see above) [24, 25, 44].

Cardiac output

Perhaps the first published study quantifying contrast echocardiography using videodensitometry was performed using a hand-held analog photoelectric cell held to a video screen over the right ventricular image [45]. In 35 patients the 50% and 90% videodensity decay times in the right ventricle correlated roughly with cardiac output. A subsequent study by the same investigators used more advanced videodensitometric analysis and 30 micron diameter plastic microballoons in a canine model with varied cardiac output. Again, a rough correlation between total area under the curve and thermodilution cardiac output was obtained (overall r = 0.65, correlation coefficients in individual dogs from r = 0.90 to 0.97) [46].

Most of the comments about limitations of videodensitometry made above apply to this technique. On the other hand, it is simple and uses no more hardware than available on most currently marketed echocardiographic instruments. If better bolus injection techniques (external jugular pushes?) and more reproducible contrast agents become available, it is quite possible that this method of cardiac output quantification may enter clinical practice.

Another quantitative contrast echocardiographic method has been proposed for the quantification of cardiac output. If the amplitude of a strong echo can be measured before and during the passage of a bolus of a known amount of ultrasonic contrast agent between the transducer and the structure, a sort of indicator-dilution curve can be constructed by the amount that the amplitude is decreased during the contrast transit. In theory, both this as well as the steady-state decrease in initial amplitude that would be seen after a constant infusion of a known amount of contrast can be used to quantify cardiac output [47]. This method has not been used for clinical studies, and our current opinion is that it is more cumbersome than the bolus method described by DeMaria and Bommer above [45, 46]. However, if the lack of bolus injection kinetics becomes the limiting problem after improvements of contrast agents and videodensitometric techniques, it is possible that the steady state – constant infusion technique might then prove useful.

Other applications

Videodensitometry has been used to quantify aortic regurgitation in an animal model using analysis of the aortic and left ventricular time-activity curves after aortic root injections [48]. This approach is interesting for theoretical reasons, but since it is invasive it offers little or no advantage over standard catheterization techniques. A problem in the use of contrast echocardiography and videodensitometry for the quantification of valvular regurgitation is that more information can be derived from injections distal to the regurgitant valve. Indicator-dilution experience has shown only limited utility gained by analysis of curves after injections proximal to the regurgitant valve [49], which would always be the case after intravenous injection. Further, problems of bolus delivery of contrast to the heart after peripheral injection also are unsolved and would contribute to the inaccuracy of videodensitometric contrast echo techniques based on venous injections.

The current effort to develop 'mini-microbubble' contrast agents capable of capillary transit would aid the diagnosis of mitral and aortic regurgitation. This could occur after IV injection if left heart contrast were attained, in a manner exactly analogous to right heart contrast echocardiographic diagnosis of tricuspid and pulmonary insufficiency [16, 17]. Further, peripheral ultrasonic arteriography of the carotids and all other arteries would be greatly aided if arterial contrast could be obtained after intravenous injections. Another medical area to benefit from improved quantitative microbubble technology, especially microbubble monitors, is the study of decompression disease. Further, quantitative ultrasonic microbubble resonance techniques may lead to noninvasive pressure measurements, though these are still in the early experimental stage at present [47, 50].

Conclusion

Quantitative contrast echocardiography is a field in its infancy that is rapidly growing and holds promise for providing practicing cardiologists with useful physiologic information in a safe and cost-effective manner, using instrumentation already widely available. These techniques are currently almost entirely experimental, however, and further clinical experience is necessary to determine their accuracy and utility. Also, much more extensive toxicity testing will be necessary before most of these techniques can be applied clinically.

References

1. Gramiak R, Shah PM: Echocardiography of the aortic root. Invest Radiol 1968; 3: 356–66.
2. Seward JB, Tajik AJ, Hagler DJ, Ritter DG: Peripheral venous contrast echocardiography. Am J Cardiol 1977; 39: 202–12.
3. Sahn DJ, Allen HD, George W, Mason M, Goldberg SJ: The utility of contrast echocardiographic techniques in the care of critically ill infants with cardiac and pulmonary disease. Circulation 1977; 56: 599–603.
4. Meltzer RS, Roelandt J (eds): Contrast Echocardiography. The Hague: Martinus Nijhoff, 1982.
5. Nanda N: Contrast echocardiography. In: Yu PN, Goodwin JF (eds): Progress in Cardiology. Philadelphia: Lea & Febiger, 1979: 133–45.
6. Corday E, Shah PN, Meerbaum S (guest editors): Seminar on contrast two-dimensional echocardiography. J Am Coll Cardiol 3: 1–5 & ff., 1984–5.
7. Meltzer RS, Vered Z, Roelandt J, Neufeld HN: Systematic analysis of contrast echocardiograms. Am J Cardiol 1983; 52: 375–80.

8. Lieppe W, Behar VS, Scallion R, Kisslo JA: Detection of tricuspid regurgitation with two-dimensional echocardiography and peripheral vein injections. Circulation 1978; 57: 128–33.

9. Meltzer RS, van Hoogenhuyze DCA, Serruys PW, Haalebos MMP, Hugenholtz PG, Roelandt J: The diagnosis of tricuspid regurgitation by contrast echocardiography. Circulation 1981; 63: 1093–99.

10. Wise NK, Meyers S, Fraker TD, Steward JA, Kisslo JA: Contrast M-mode ultrasonography of the inferior vena cava. Circulation 1981; 63: 1100–1103.

11. Levin AR, Spach MS, Canent RV, Boineau JP, Capp MP, Jain V, Barr RC: Intracardiac pressure-flow dynamics in isolated ventricular septal defects. Circulation 1967; 35: 430–41.

12. Serwer GA, Armstrong BE, Anderson PAW, Sherman D, Benson W, Edwards SB: Use of contrast echocardiography for evaluation of right ventricular hemodynamics in the presence of ventricular septal defects. Circulation 1978; 58: 327–36.

13. Kronik G: Contrast echocardiography in patent foramen ovale. In: Meltzer RS, Roelandt J (eds): Contrast Echocardiography. The Hague: Martinus Nijhoff, 1982: 137–52.

14. Mortera C, Hunter S, Tynan M: Contrast echocardiography and the suprasternal approach in infants and children. Eur J Cardiol 1979; 9: 437–54.

15. Tsuyuguchi N, Nohara R, Suwo M, Yoshimatsu S, Tamagawa M, Shigeta H, Hashimoto M, Kaneko R: Evaluation of cardiac function by contrast echo disappearance time. J Cardiography 1981; 11: 467–75.

16. Meltzer RS, Vered Z, Benjamin P, Hegesh J, Visser CA, Neufeld HN: Diagnosing tricuspid regurgitation by direct imaging of the regurgitant flow in the right atrium using contrast echocardiography. Am J Cardiol 1983; 52: 1050–53.

17. Meltzer RS, Vered Z, Hegesh J, Benjamin P. Visser CA, Shem-Tov A, Neufeld HN: Diagnosis of pulmonic regurgitation by contrast echocardiography. Am Heart 1984; 107: 102–7.

18. Levine RA, Teichholz LE, Goldman ME, Steinmetz MY, Baker M, Meltzer RS: Microbubbles have intracardiac velocities similar to red blood cells. J Am Coll Cardiol 1984; 3: 28–33.

19. Zeiher AM, Bonzel T, Wollschlager H, Just J: Diagnostic value of quantitative contrast M-mode echocardiography at the pulmonary valve. Submitted to J Am Coll Cardiol.

20. Feinstein SB, ten Cate FJ, Zwehl W, Ong K, Maurer G, Tei C, Shah PM, Meerbaum S, Corday E: Two dimensional contrast echocardiography. I. In vitro development and quantitative analysis of echo contrast agents. J Am Coll Cardiol 1984; 3: 14–20.

21. Smith MD, Kwan OL, Reiser HJ, DeMaria AN: Superior intensity and reproducibility of SHU-454, a new right heart contrast agent. J Am Coll Cardiol 1984; 3: 992–8.

22. Meltzer RS, Klig V, Teichholz LE: Generating precision microbubbles for use as an echocardiographic contrast agent. J Am Coll Cardiol 1985; 5: 978–82.

23. Meltzer RS, Koenig K, Klig V, Teichholz LE: Effect of viscosity on the size of microbubbles generated for use as echo contrast agents. Submitted to the American Heart Association, 58th scientific session, (abstract).

24. Zwehl W, Areeda J, Schwartz G, Feinstein S, Ong K, Meerbaum S: Physical factors influencing quantitation of two-dimensional contrast echo amplitudes. J Am Coll Cardiol 1984; 4: 157–64.

25. Ong K, Maurer G, Feinstein S, Zwehl W, Meerbaum S, Corday E: Computer methods for myocardial contrast two-dimensional echocardiography. J Am Coll Cardiol 1984; 3: 1212–8.

26. DeMaria AN, Bommer WJ, Riggs K et al.: Echocardiographic visualization of myocardial perfusion by left heart and intracoronary injections of echo contrast agent. Circulation 1980; 60 (Suppl. III): III–143 (abstract).

27. Armstrong W, Mueller T, Kinney E, Thickner G, Dillon J, Feigenbaum H: Assessment of myocardial perfusion abnormalities with contrast enhanced two-dimensional echocardiography. Circulation 1982; 66: 166–74.

28. Meltzer RS, Vermeulen HW, Valk N, Verdouw P, Lancee CT, Roelandt J: New echocardiographic contrast agents: transmission through the lungs and myocardial perfusion imaging. J Cardiovasc Ultrasonography 1982; 1: 277–82.

29. Goldman ME, Mindich BP: Intraoperative cardioplegic contrast echocardiography for assessing

myocardial perfusion during open heart surgery. J Am Coll Cardiol 1984; 5: 1029–34.

30. Santoso T, Roelandt J, Mansjoer H, Abdurahman M, Meltzer RS, Hugenholtz PG: Use of polygelin colloid solution for contrast echocardiographic myocardial perfusion imaging in humans. J Am Coll Cardiol (in press).

31. Sakamaki T, Tei C, Meerbaum S, Shimoura K, Kondo S, Fishbein MC, Y-Rit J, Shah PM, Corday E: Verification of myocardial contrast two-dimensional echocardiographic assessment of perfusion defects in ischemic myocardium. J Am Coll Cardiol 1984; 3: 34–8.

32. Tei C, Kondo S, Meerbaum S, Ong K, Maurer G, Wood F, Sakamaki T, Shimoura K, Corday E, Shah PM: Correlation of myocardial echo contrast disappearance rate ('washout') and severity of experimental coronary stenosis. J Am Coll Cardiol 1984; 3: 39–46.

33. Ten Cate FJ, Drury JK, Meerbaum S, Noordsy J, Feinstein S, Shah PM: Myocardial contrast two-dimensional echocardiography: experimental examination at different coronary flow levels. J Am Coll Cardiol 1984; 3: 1219–26.

34. Kondo S, Tei C, Meerbaum S, Corday E, Shah PM: Hyperemic response of intracoronary contrast agents during two-dimensional echographic delineation of regional myocardium. J Am Coll Cardiol 1984; 4: 149–56.

35. Bommer WJ, Shah PM, Allen H, Meltzer R, Kisslo J: The safety of contrast echocardiography: report of the committee on contrast echocardiography for the American Society of Echocardiography. J Am Coll Cardiol 1984; 3: 6–13.

36. Gillam LD, Kaul S, Fallon JT, Hedley-White ET, Slater CE, Weyman AE: Sequelae of echocardiographic contrast: studies of myocardium, brain, and kidney. Circulation 1984; 70 (Suppl. II): II–6 (abstract).

37. Holt G, Reeves W, Rieder M, Daley L, Murthy V, Christensen C: Negative inotropic effects of intracoronary echo-contrast agents. J Am Coll Cardiol 1985; 5: 474 (abstract).

38. Levine RA, Gillam LD, Guerrero JL, Weyman AE: Wall motion abnormalities following myocardial echo contrast injection are caused by microbubbles. J Am Coll Cardiol 1985; 5: 474 (abstract).

39. Hagler DJ, Tajik AJ, Seward JB, Mair DD, Ritter DG, Ritman EL: Videodensitometric quantitation of left-to-right shunts with contrast sector echocardiography. Circulation 1978; 58 (Suppl. II): II–70 (abstract).

40. Hagler DJ, Tajik AJ, Seward JB, Ritman EL, in: Meltzer RS, Roelandt J (eds): Contrast Echocardiography. The Hague: Martinus Nijhoff, 1982: 298–303.

41. Serwer GA, Armstrong BE, Anderson PAW, Sherman D, Benson DW, Edwards SB: Use of contrast echocardiography for evaluation of right ventricular hemodynamics in the presence of ventricular septal defects. Circulation 1978; 58: 327.

42. Serwer GA, Armstrong BE: Contrast echocardiography for evaluation of right ventricular hemodynamics in the presence of ventricular septal defects. In: Meltzer RS, Roelandt J (eds): Contrast Echocardiography. The Hague: Martinus Nijhoff, 1982: 179–91.

43. Valdes-Cruz LM, Sahn DJ: Ultrasonic contrast studies for the detection of cardiac shunts. J Am Coll Cardiol 1984; 3: 978–85.

44. Meltzer RS, Bastiaans OL, Lancee CT, Pierard L, Serruys PW, Roelandt J: Videodensitometric processing of contrast two-dimensional echocardiographic data. Ultrasound in Med & Biol 1982; 8: 509–14.

45. Bommer WJ, Neef J, Neuman A, Weinert L, Lee G, Mason DT, DeMaria AN: Indicator-dilution curves obtained by photometric analysis of two-dimensional echo-contrast studies. Am J Cardiol 1978; 41: 370 (abstract).

46. DeMaria AN, Bommer W, Kwan OL, Riggs K, Smith M, Waters J: In vivo correlation of thermodilution cardiac output and videodensitometric indicator-dilution curves obtained from contrast two-dimensional echocardiograms. J Am Coll Cardiol 1984; 3: 999–1004.

47. Tickner EG: Precision microbubbles for right-sided intracardiac pressure and flow measurements. In: Meltzer RS, Roelandt J (eds): Contrast Echocardiography. The Hague: Martinus Nijhoff, 1982: 313–24.

58

48. Sahn DJ, Valdes-Cruz LM, Jones M, Main J, Swensson RE, Elias W, Eidbo E, Gerber KH: Contrast echocardiographic quantitation of aortic insufficiency: studies in an animal model using a standardized experimental echo contrast agent. J Am Coll Cardiol 1984; 3: 563 (abstract).
49. Bloomfield DA (ed), Dye Curves. Baltimore: University Park Press, 1974.
50. Prof. VL Newhouse, Philadelphia, PA – personnal communication.

Part Two: Tissue Characterization

6. Quantitative Acoustic Characterization of the Myocardium*

Robert H. HOYT[1], Steve M. COLLINS[2] and David J. SKORTON[2]
[1] University of Arizona, USA, [2] University of Iowa, USA

Background

Quantitative ultrasonic analysis of the myocardium for non-invasive medical diagnosis is based on the premise that alterations in acoustic properties of the myocardium accompany the development of myocardial disease. Implicit in this approach is knowledge of the acoustic properties of normal myocardium. Also required is ultrasonic and computer instrumentation capable of quantifying one or more acoustic parameters, and interfacing with existing clinical echocardiographic equipment. Both M-mode and two-dimensional (2D) echocardiography utilize specular reflection to depict smooth tissue interfaces such as the pericardium, epicardium, endocardium, valve leaflets, and aortic root. Although not designed for the purpose of tissue characterization, standard echocardiographic systems have yielded a variety of qualitative imaging observations in human hearts that underscore the potential clinical importance of quantitative characterization of the myocardium (Table 1) [1–8]. Common to most of the disease

Table 1. Qualitative echocardiographic observations of abnormal myocardium.

Tissue diagnosis	Echo pattern	Reference
Myocardial scar	Multiple bands of increased echogenicity	[1]
	Highly refractile echoes >5 mm	[7]
Infiltrative cardiomyopathy	Highly refractile echoes 3–5 mm	[7]
Hypertrophic cardiomyopathy	Ground glass texture	[2]
Endocardial fibroelastosis	High intensity and layering of endocardial echoes	[3, 5]
Amyloidosis	Granular sparkling	[4]
Intracardiac masses	Uniform speckling, lucency, bright echoes	[6]

* Supported in part by: Specialized Center for Research (SCOR) Grant in Ischemic Heart Disease 1-P50-HL32295 and Research Career Development Award K04HL01290 (Dr. Skorton) from the U.S.P.H.S., National Institutes of Health, and the F.E. Rippel Foundation.

J. Roelandt (editor), Digital Techniques in Echocardiography. ISBN 0-89838-861-9.

processes listed in Table 1 is replacement of the normal myocardium by tissue elements (amyloid, calcium, collagen) likely to have different acoustic properties than the surrounding myocardium. The irregular shape of these elements leads to scattering rather than specular reflection of incident ultrasound.

Instrument-related factors influencing quantitative characterization

Instrumentation for tissue characterization studies employing radio frequency data analysis usually includes a computer-based data acquisition system with capability for rapid high resolution analog to digital conversion (fast transient recorder), spectral analysis, and electronic gating (Figure 1). Processing of 2D echocardiographic images may utilize additional capabilities for real-time video digitization, digital scan conversion (from polar to rectangular display formats), and computer-based video processing, storage, and graphics [9, 10].

For tissue characterization, both narrow and broadband transducers with a wide range of center frequencies (2–25 MHz) have been employed by various investigators. From a theoretical standpoint, a broadband transducer is advantageous since data may be derived on the frequency dependence of ultrasonic parameters, and frequency averaging procedures may be performed to reduce random signal fluctuations [11]. From a practical standpoint, the intervening chest wall acts as a low-pass filter, due to increased attenuation of ultrasound by the chest wall at higher frequencies [12]. Thus, transducer center frequencies in the range of 2–5 MHz are used most commonly for diagnostic studies in adult patients.

Piezoelectric transducers (finite aperture) are subject to artifactual distortion of the incident wavefront due to the effects of acoustic inhomogeneity of the myocardium. This inhomogeneity produces a complex pattern of interference of reflections from tissue. The destructive and constructive interference effects, as detected with a piezoelectric transducer, are known as phase cancellation artifacts in the measurement of ultrasonic indices (such as attenuation or backscatter), and speckle in 2D echocardiographic images [13–15]. This artifact may be reduced by averaging a sufficient number of signals to smooth random fluctuations. For attenuation applications, a cadmium sulfide receiving element based on the acoustoelectric effect has been demonstrated to eliminate phase cancellation effects [14]. For speckle reduction in 2D images, transducer and instrument modifications such as parallel focusing and multiple frequency arrays, have been introduced [15, 16].

Quantitative indices of both unprocessed radio frequency signals and envelope-detected video data exhibit a wide dynamic range; thus quantitation is facilitated by decibel notation. A decibel (dB) is 10 times the logarithm of a power or energy (intensity) ratio, or 20 times the logarithm of a voltage or current (amplitude) ratio. For convenience in interpretation of ultrasonic data, Table 2

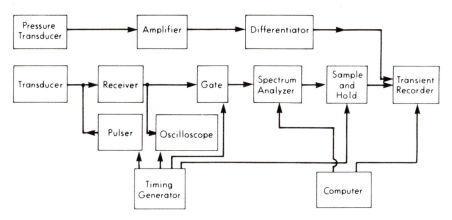

Fig. 1. Diagram of a data acquisition system for ultrasonic tissue characterization (reproduced from reference 22 with permission of the author and the American Heart Association, Inc.).

relates decibel change to percent change in signal intensity. The dynamic range of pulsed ultrasound in its radio frequency form is on the order of 100 dB; video detection compresses this into a gray scale display of approximately 20–40 dB, tending to obscure gradations in regional echo amplitude. The digital signal processing required to generate 2D echocardiographic images introduces additional error by nonlinear amplitude compression, envelope detection, thresholding, and position of the region of interest within the scan field [17]. Another important source of acoustic variability in 2D echocardiograms is the method of gain compensation for attenuation. Melton and Skorton have devised one system, termed 'rational gain compensation', which accounts for differences in attenuation by intervening tissue or blood along each scan line of a 2D echocardiogram [18]. Other methods, such as that of O'Donnell, have also been introduced to account for attenuation of ultrasound by tissue interposed between the transducer and region of interest [19]. Quantitative measures in 2D echocardiography, such as mean regional gray level or texture analysis, are subject to all these artifacts. The specific processing-induced differences in the relationship between analog radio frequency data and echo amplitude (video) data vary among equipment manufacturers.

Table 2. Decibel scale.

Decibel change	% increase (intensity ratio)
0.41	10
1.76	50
3.01	100
5.0	216
7.0	401
10.0	900

Tissue-related factors influencing quantitative characterization

Investigation of the ultrasonic characteristics of the heart has lagged somewhat behind that of other organs (such as the eye, breast, or liver) that are stationary and accessible targets. Cardiac ultrasonic data acquisition in vivo is performed via limited views through the intercostal spaces. Cardiovascular dynamics (the translational, rotational, and contractile motion of the heart), as well as respiratory movements, hinder the performance of ultrasonic studies. As a result of these motions, the myocardial region of interest constantly changes depth and orientation with respect to a transducer in a fixed position on the chest wall. This may lead to artifactual alterations in echo amplitudes due to changes of both the position of the insonified sample volume within the heart and the attenuation profile between the region of interest and the transducer. Such movement may also lead to sampling error when tissue is later removed from a specific region of interest for histologic or biochemical analysis.

Early in vivo studies of attenuation and backscatter measured echo data that was averaged through the cardiac cycle. It is easily conceptualized that contractile changes in left ventricular wall thickness known to occur through the cardiac cycle might influence the position and content of the sample volume, as well as the density, and geometric relationship of ultrasonic scatterers. An in vivo study of open chest dogs by O'Donnell et al. alludes to this finding [11]. Subsequently Madaras, Barzilai, and co-workers developed a gating system comprised of a series of seven 34 msec windows, each separated by 18 msec, to describe the cyclic variation of myocardial ultrasonic backscatter [20, 21]. This technique was subsequently expanded to sample 32 different windows through the cardiac cycle [22]. Such cycle timed sampling procedures reduce error caused by contractile motion of the heart.

When evaluating studies that attempt to correlate regional ultrasonic quantities to histologic or biochemical measures, the method of verifying that a tissue sample is actually excised from the appropriate ultrasonic region of interest is important. In published studies, this has varied from a subjective judgement of the approximate location and orientation of the insonifying beam, to spearing the region of interest with an echo-directed needle passed through the chest, to carefully defined sample volumes based upon considerations of beam width, orientation, and range-gated sample thickness [23–25].

Furthermore, myocardial disease processes, such as ischemia, are more often than not heterogeneous within a given region of interest for ultrasonic study. This is illustrated in an early study by Gramiak et al. relating B-scan echo amplitudes to the identification of acute myocardial infarction in dog hearts [23]. Infarct zones were demarcated by intravenous thioflavin S, which upon postmortem study demonstrated perfusion deficits without reference to the degree of underperfusion within the infarct risk area. This led to the conclusion that ultrasound frequently underestimates infarct size, and was subject to a high rate of false positive and false negative results. Subsequently, Mimbs et al. evaluated ultra-sonic backscatter in the same animal model [26]. The degree of ischemia was quantitated by ^{141}Ce microspheres, and was found to vary within the infarct risk areas. Ultrasonic measures were then shown to correspond closely with acute ischemia in regions with less than 20% of control blood flow, presumably com-mitted to irreversible injury [26].

Additional considerations relate to whether the entire thickness of the ven-tricular free wall (between epi- and endocardial specular reflections) is assessed ultrasonically, since many studies have gated signals from only midwall segments of myocardium [12, 21]. This is important since myocardial disease may be preferentially located with respect to the epi- and endocardium (such as epicar-dial fatty infiltration or subendocardial ischemia). A small portion of the sub-epicardial mantle is lost during 'ringing down' of the epicardial specular echo. Only the compact portion of the free wall can be reliably studied with tissue characterization methods, since the convolved trabeculae of the endocardial layer give rise to angle dependent specular reflections [25].

Finally, in vitro determinations of ultrasonic indices may be influenced by tissue temperature, and the time interval between loss of tissue viability and study [27, 28]. Fixation techniques may overcome this latter problem. Formalin fixation of myocardium is a convenient method of preservation for later in vitro study, and does not appear to significantly alter left ventricular ultrasonic backscatter com-pared to the freshly excised state [25].

Quantitative methods

Techniques proposed for quantitative characterization of the myocardium may be divided into two broad categories: 1) direct measurement or analysis of regional one-dimensional ultrasonic radio frequency data, 2) detection of myo-cardial disease by digital analysis of 2D echocardiograms.

One-dimensional analysis

Ultrasonic indices which may be measured directly in myocardial tissue include velocity, acoustic impedance, attenuation, and scattering (Table 3). Since these parameters depend on the intrinsic physical properties of the tissue, they may be likened to a pathologic examination in which changes in the palpatory character of the tissue is used to infer the presence of specific disease processes; for example, softening suggests acute infarction and stiffening implies fibrosis. These indices are usually assessed with the ultrasonic transducer oriented perpendicular to the myocardial region of interest, to unambiguously demonstrate the surface specular reflection and avoid fluctuations in echo amplitude dependent on orientation [29]. The surface specular reflection is positioned near the focal length of a planar transducer to utilize the smooth sound field intensity pattern of the far field; or the focal zone of a focused transducer may be used for data acquisition.

Acoustic velocity (c) is a function of the elasticity (compressibility or inverse of bulk modulus) of the myocardium. Shung and Reid have developed the following method for in vitro determination of velocity: a segment of myocardium is inserted between two aluminum rods, ant the time interval (T_1) between echoes from each aluminum/myocardial interface is noted [28]. The myocardium is removed, and the time of propagation of ultrasound through an equivalent distance of saline (T_2) is also measured. The velocity of ultrasound in saline $(c_1,$ approximately 1,490 msec) is used to derive the velocity in myocardium (c_2) by the proportion: $c_2 = (T_1)(c_1)/T_2$.

Acoustic impedance is a product of the density of myocardium and the acoustic velocity. Namery and Lele assessed impedance of the myocardium in vitro using A-scan, by comparison to targets of known acoustic impedance such as glass, plexiglass, and polyethylene [29]. Gregg and Palagallo also used a polyethylene reference medium impedance $(\varrho c)_1$ and derived a value for impedance of the myocardium $(\varrho c)_2$ by the formula: $(\varrho c)_2 = (\varrho c)_1 (1-V_r/V+V_r)$; V_r is the ratio of specular reflection amplitudes of the two media [30].

Attenuation refers to loss of energy occurring as ultrasound propagates through the myocardium [31]. This may occur as a consequence of absorption or scattering (see below), and appears to be related to frequency dependent interactions of ultrasound with macromolecular and cellular constituents of the myocardium [32]. Measurements usually have been obtained using separate transmitting and receiving elements placed on either side of the tissue specimen. Thus attenuation data are of limited potential for application in clinical echocardiography, since there are no transthoracic portals for ultrasonic transmission. Attenuation may be quantitated by comparison of the signal loss occurring with transmission

Table 3. Quantitative indices.

Parameter	Equation	Symbols	Reference
Velocity (c)	$C = \sqrt{1/\varrho\beta}$	β: compressibility ϱ: density	[31]
Acoustic impedance (Z)	$Z = \varrho c = \sqrt{\varrho K}$	K: bulk modulus	[30, 31]
Attenuation (decrease in intensity [1])	$I(z) = I_o e^{-(\mu_a+\mu_s)z}$	μ_a: absorption coefficient μ_s: scattering coefficient z: depth	[31]
Integrated backscatter ($\check{S}$)	$\check{S} = \dfrac{\int_{-\infty}^{\infty} \lvert a(t)\rvert^2 dt}{\int_{-\infty}^{\infty} \lvert p(t)\rvert^2 dt}$	a(t): signal from tissue p(t): signal from reference plane reflector	[11]

through a specified thickness of myocardium, to the signal transmitted through saline. Mimbs et al. used broadband (2–11 MHz) pulses for attenuation studies of the myocardium [33]. The transmitted pulse was gated into an analog spectrum analyzer and subjected to Fourier analysis. An attenuation coefficient was calculated and plotted as a function of frequency. The slope of the best fit line to this plot was used as an index of attenuation.

Ultrasonic scattering may be described as low level echoes originating between the specular reflections that identify the epicardium and endocardium. This process results from the effects on wave propagation of acoustic inhomogeneity of the myocardium [31, 34]. As in the case of attenuation, such 'inhomogeneities' appear to be determined in part by interaction between ultrasound and myocardial cellular constituents at the macromolecular, cellular, and macroscopic levels [35]. Such interactions reflect local variations in myocardial density, compressibility, and viscosity; as well as the size, shape, and geometrical distribution of scatterers [36]. Backscatter is the portion of scattered energy returning along the path of the incident wavefront. The backscattered wave is a composite interference pattern of the phase-front disturbances occurring with propagation of ultrasound in the myocardium. Backscattering from the myocardium increases as a function of frequency (2–10 MHz) by a third power dependence (Figure 2) [28]. Shung and Reid have pointed out, considering the theory of wave scattering by small cylinders, that this relationship suggests the size of scatterers in the normal myocardium is less than $20 \, \mu m$, approximately twice the diameter of normal cardiac muscle fibers [28].

Since backscatter can be detected by reflection-based instrumentation, it appears to be the most clinically applicable of the regional ultrasonic indices. M-mode recordings are not designed to display these low level echoes. In 2D echocardiographic images, backscatter accounts in part for the variegated gray levels, or texture, observed within the myocardium. The potential for obtaining backscatter measurements with existing clinical devices is demonstrated by the investigational use of M-mode and 2D equipment to access unprocessed radio frequency backscatter waveforms, prior standard display modifications [37, 38].

Theoretical analysis of the physical basis underlying the scattering process has yielded several approaches for quantification of backscatter in the time and frequency domains [39]. First, the backscatter coefficient is defined as the differential scattering cross section per unit solid angle for 180° scattering [40]. It is derived from the ratio of the Fourier-transformed backscatter signal from tissue, to that from a plane reflector substituted for the tissue. Second, the integrated backscatter (Table 3) is the frequency average of a backscatter transfer function over the bandwidth of the transducer [11]. The transfer function is proportional to the area under the power spectrum of the radio frequency backscatter signal. This parameter is particularly applicable to in vivo tissue characterization, since it may be measured simply as the energy of the backscatter signal from a discrete (spatially localized) volume of tissue relative to the energy of a reference specular

68

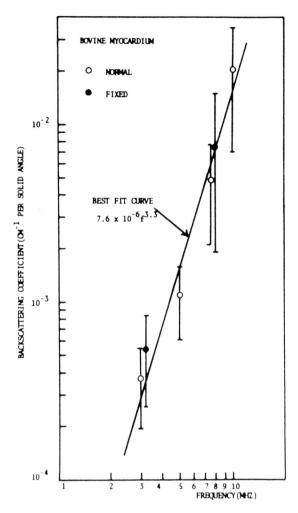

Fig. 2. Backscattering from the myocardium increases as a function of frequency by a third power dependence (reproduced from reference 28 with permission of the author and the IEEE).

echo. Because of the frequency-averaging procedure, information about the frequency dependence of scattering is lost. A third approach, proposed by Joynt and collaborators, is based upon stochastic models of ultrasound interaction with tissue [41]. This may include measures such as a coefficient (k) describing the degree of departure of the distribution of regional echo amplitudes from that predicted by a Rayleigh distribution [37]. This digital signal analysis method has the advantage of providing a variety of statistical measures of the backscattered waveform independent of equipment parameters and the effects of intervening tissues. A potential disadvantage of such an empirical approach may be the lack of a specific understanding of the underlying mechanisms by which alterations of tissue structure may influence specific statistical measures.

Two-dimensional analysis

The intramural gray level patterns observed in 2D echocardiographic studies depends on backscatter, attenuation plus phase cancellation effects, and the process of digital image generation. The inherent spatial resolution of pulsed ultrasound has led to the general practice of image projection into a 128^2 or 256^2 pixel (picture element) matrix. Each pixel is then assigned one of a range of gray levels from white to black, corresponding to the echo intensity associated with that pixel. Commercially available digital echocardiographs may provide up to 8 bit or 256 gray level quantization.

As previously described, the reports of distinct intramural echo patterns observed in the 2D echocardiograms of patients with myocardial disease suggest important diagnostic information may be present in such patterns. Unfortunately, these observations have been sporadic and nonspecific, owing in part to difficulties in accurate perception of altered gray levels. Pseudocolor encoding of the gray scale display format represents an attempt to enhance perception by the human eye of regional echo gray level differences in a semiquantitative manner. Generally, gray levels are segmented stepwise into one of eight levels, each of which is assigned a color. The color spectrum chosen to represent each gradation has varied among authors and the manufacturers of color display equipment. This technique has facilitated somewhat the ability of trained observers to recognize various types of myocardial disease, including experimental infarction in dogs, as well as cardiac tumors and fibrosis in patients [42–44).

Quantitative measures of gray level patterns in 2D echocardiograms have been approached in various ways. One method is simply to determine the average gray level within a particular region of interest [45]. This is analogous to a video processed version of the regional backscatter amplitude. Two-dimensional echo data also lends itself to empirical study in a manner analogous to the stochastic analysis of backscatter discussed previously. For example, regional echo patterns may be analyzed by the shape (e.g., skewness or kurtosis) of gray level histograms denoting the frequency of occurrence of pixels at each particular gray level within the region of interest [45, 46].

A potentially more specific approach is the use of quantitative texture analysis [47]. Texture may be defined as the two-dimensional distribution or spatial pattern of echo amplitudes. Thus, two regions might have the same average gray level, but distinctly different textures (Figure 3). Quantitation of texture involves a statistical measure of image detail such as run length, edge count, entropy, or gray level differences. For example, a run length is based on the concept of a set of consecutive pixels having the same gray level, or gray level values within a specified range. These may be assessed by measures emphasizing long or short runs, run-length nonuniformity, or run percentage. Each calculation may be performed in one or more directions for a specified region of interest.

An approach relating integrated backscatter, as opposed to the envelope

70

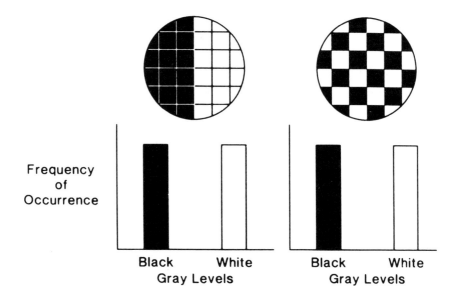

Fig. 3. Texture analysis quantifies the spatial distribution of echo amplitudes. The two diagrams illustrate regions of interest with the same histogram distribution of gray levels, but a distinct difference in texture (reproduced from reference 47 with permission of the author and the American Heart Association, Inc.).

detected signal, to a 2D imaging format has been developed by Rasmussen et al. [38]. These investigators used an off-line computer system to access and directly digitize unprocessed analog 2D echocardiographic signals. Echo intensities were used to calculate an integrated backscatter ratio (with reference to the specular reflection at the posterior left ventricular endocardial boundary) for 480 points along each scan line. These points were used to draw echo intensity contour maps and determine integrated backscatter ratios within specific regions of interest.

Acoustic properties of normal and abnormal myocardium

Normal myocardium

The velocity of ultrasound propagation through normal myocardium has been measured at 1570 m/sec [48]. Gregg and Palagallo obtained an acoustic impedance of $1.64 \pm 0.3 \times 10^5$ g/cm$^2 \div$sec in normal human left ventricle obtained at autopsy; and in a dog heart found a modest decline in the impedance of postmortem compared to in vivo left ventricular myocardium [30].

Attenuation varies throughout the normal left ventricle, being highest in the papillary muscle and lowest at the base (Figure 4) [27]. O'Donnell et al. reported an attenuation coefficient in excised dog left ventricle of approximately 0.19 cm^{-1}

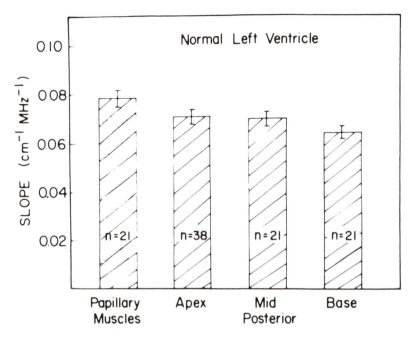

Fig. 4. Ultrasonic attenuation exhibits regional variation within the left ventricle, with higher values found in the papillary muscles than in basilar segments (reproduced from reference 27 with permission of the author and the publisher).

[49]. Klepper and coworkers demonstrated that the slope of a line fit to the attenuation coefficient as a function of frequency ranges from 0.13–0.17 cm^{-1} MHz^{-1}, and varied with the projection angle of ultrasound incident upon an excised segment of left ventricle [13]. This dependence of attenuation on angle of the insonifying beam to the specimen indicates that acoustic anisotropy is a characteristic of normal myocardium. This finding was confirmed by Mottley and Miller [50], and is true of skeletal muscle as well [51]. Anisotropy may be attributed to myocardial muscle fiber organization. Normal left ventricular myocardium is comprised of inner and outer spiral and deep constrictor layers, which interdigitate and subtend varying oblique angles with respect to the dominant fiber orientation in the adjacent layer. In a general sense, anisotropy is a factor which may account for some regional variations in ultrasonic indices.

A second factor which may contribute to regional variation in acoustic properties is the local concentration of collagen, which is known to be higher in the right than left ventricle of many species [52, 53]. Hoyt et al. found a 4.9 dB increase in the 2.25 MHz integrated backscatter in the right ventricle compared to the left ventricle of normal formalin-fixed human hearts, which was associated with a 30% higher collagen concentration in the right ventricle (Figure 5) [25]. Backscatter amplitudes tended to be uniform from epi- to endocardium. Information concerning the relationship between the average backscatter and location within

72

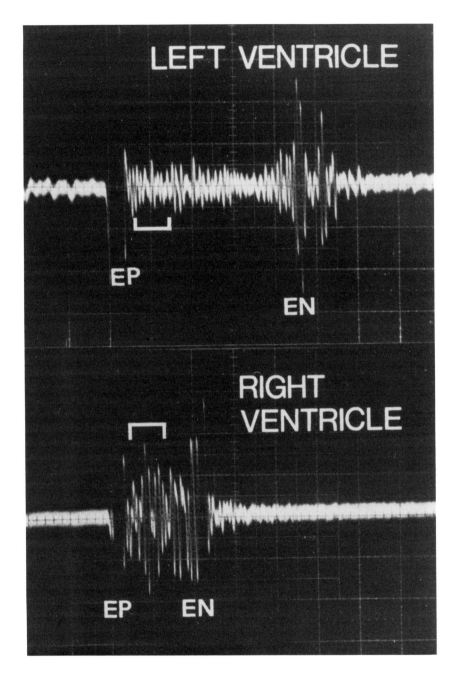

Fig. 5. Unprocessed radio frequency backscatter signal (2.25 MHz) from normal human ventricles in vitro. The average level of backscatter within a 4 μsec gate (brackets) is higher in the right than in the left ventricle. Endocardial (EN) echoes are often multiple and appear to correspond to trabeculation (calibration: 5 μsec/div. horizontal, 0.5 mV/div. vertical, EP = epicardial interface), (reproduced from reference 25 with permission of the author and the American Heart Association, Inc.).

the left ventricle suggest no differences from apex to base, or between the midwall ventricular septum compared to the mid-anterior left ventricular free wall [22, 54]. Cohen et al. suggested the attenuation effects of pericardial fat were minimal and had little influence on backscatter measurements [12].

Few tissue characterization data are yet available concerning the normal atria. Baello et al. found that atrial backscatter was higher than backscatter from corresponding ventricles in normal, perfusion-fixed dog hearts [55]; this follows the known pattern fo collagen distribution [56].

In vivo studies of canine myocardium indicate that integrated backscatter fluctuates by an average of 3.5 dB (124% change) through the cardiac cycle, being highest at end-diastole and lowest at end-systole (Figure 6) [20]. The degree of this amplitude fluctuation is regionally dependent, varying from only 0.5 dB in basilar segments to 5.5 dB in apical segments [22]. In asynchronously paced or propranolol treated dogs, Wickline et al. suggested that local contractile performance is the major determinant of this cyclic variation in backscatter [57]. There was also 50% greater amplitude of cyclic variation in subendocardial than subepicardial areas. Olshansky et al. noted analogous cyclic fluctuations of left ventricular gray levels in 2D echocardiograms; however, the maximal change was on the order of 20% [58]. This may be accounted for by the sampling of echo amplitudes from the posterobasal left ventricular region of the 2D image. A comparable (0.5 dB or 12%) amplitude of cyclic variation in the integrated backscatter from basilar segments was reported by Madaras [20]. This suggests a degree of correspondence between levels of integrated backscatter (currently an investigational method) and the video-detected echo amplitude, which is clinically applicable. Recent studies of quantitative echocardiographic texture analysis also demonstrated a cardiac cycle-dependent variation in image texture [59].

Logan-Sinclair and associates evaluated regional 2D echo amplitudes referenced to the posterior pericardial/lung specular reflection in 20 normal human subjects [42]. The central fibrous body had the highest echo amplitude (64 ± 5% [SD]). The echo intensity of the ventricular septum (33 ± 8%) was greater than the posterior wall of the left ventricle (23 ± 6%, p<0.05); however no attempts were made to account for possible attenuation differences along the transducer line-of-sight between these regions [42]. In pre-infarction control 2D images from seven normal dog hearts which were corrected for background gray level differences, Skorton et al. found no significant difference in the average gray level obtained from the anterolateral wall, posterior wall, and ventricular septum [45]. Haendchen et al. studied average pixel intensity in normal pre-infarction control regions of eight dogs, and found no apparent differences between subendocardial versus subepicardial segments of the left ventricle [46]. In normal dogs, texture analysis measures do not vary significantly between the ventricular septum and anterolateral left ventricle [47]. Stochastic analysis by Schnittger et al. indicates that normal myocardium behaves in a manner similar to an ensemble of independent scatterers, leading to a characteristic Rayleigh (normal) distribution of backscatter amplitudes [24].

74

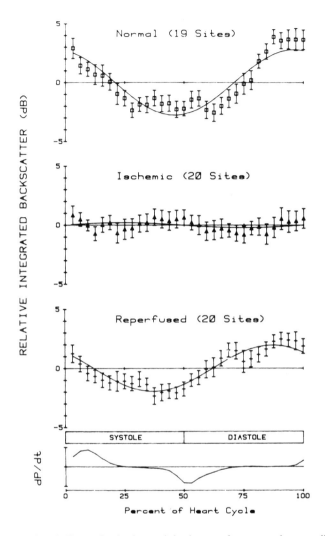

Fig. 6. Amplitude of cyclic fluctuation in ultrasonic backscatter from normal myocardium (top panel), decline after 10 minutes of ischemia (top center panel), and partial normalization after 2 hours of reperfusion (lower center panel), (reproduced from reference 22 with permission of the author and the American Heart Association, Inc.).

There have been no longitudinal studies in humans to determine the effects of normal aging on ultrasonic indices. Perez et al. reported that the 25 MHz integrated backscatter from normal hamster hearts studied at either 2–3 or 5–7 months of age increased from -58.7 ± 0.08 (SE) dB to -55.9 ± 0.11 dB respectively (p<0.05) [60]. One possible implication is that evaluations of ultrasonic indices may need to be referenced to the patient's age.

A major difficulty in use of the absolute value of integrated backscatter to differentiate normal from diseased myocardium is the wide range of values among normal left ventricles. This is typically on the order of 10 dB in dog hearts and 5 dB in human hearts [21, 25].

Ischemic heart disease

Acute myocardial infarction

Limited information is available concerning the velocity of sound in infarcted myocardium. Namery and Lele studied dogs subjected to 20–30 minutes of left circumflex coronary artery ligation, and found that excised segments demonstrated a decline in both acoustic impedance and attenuation [29].

Mimbs et al. studied in vitro 517 ischemic regions from 41 dogs following ligation of the left anterior descending (LAD) coronary artery [27]. The slope of a line fit to the frequency dependence of the attenuation coefficient over the range 2–10 MHz was approximately 0.072 cm^{-1} MHz^{-1} in non-ischemic control regions. This declined to a level of approximately 0.063 cm^{-1} MHz^{-1} at 15 min after coronary ligation, and remained essentially unchanged at 1, 6, and 24 hours postligation (Figure 7). By three days post-infarction, attenuation had actually increased compared to control values, and a further increase was observed by six weeks. Thus, quantitative alterations in ultrasonic attenuation are associated with acute and healing infarction [27].

O'Donnell et al. evaluated integrated ultrasonic backscatter averaged over six cardiac cycles with a 5 MHz broadband transducer in open chest dogs with LAD artery ligation. There was a substantial (about 3 dB) increase in the backscatter at 1 hour, reaching a plateau at 6 dB from 2–6 hours post-occlusion [11]. Mimbs et al. demonstrated that a significant increase in the backscatter occurred only in ischemic regions with less than 20% control blood flow as assessed by [141]Ce microspheres [26]. Furthermore, in 17 isolated perfused rabbit hearts, increases in backscatter of a similar magnitude could be produced by lowering the albumin concentration in the perfusate from 3% to 1% [26]. This corresponded to a rise in the wet weight of myocardium, suggesting that myocardial edema occurring early after occlusion contributes to the increased magnitude of scattering. The data of Dines et al. support this concept, indicating that myocardial fiber bundle and scatterer spacings increase after coronary ligation, providing a mechanism by which myocardial edema formation may increase scattering [61]. In addition, Rasmussen et al. suggested that increased scattering in acute infarction may result from arteriolar and capillary collapse occurring with loss of blood flow, resulting in the formation of many small reflective laminar surfaces [38].

Cohen et al. found similar differences in backscatter 2–4 hours after LAD artery occlusion, and derived a correction factor for frequency-dependent attenuation by the chest wall [12]. This correction permitted close approximation of backscatter measurements in open and closed chest dogs for both control and ischemic sites. Even without the correction factor, it is evident from these data

76

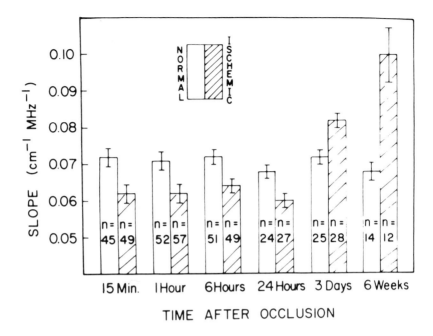

Fig. 7. The index of ultrasonic attenuation, shown on the ordinate, is decreased within 15 minutes of coronary occlusion, then increases from 3 days to 6 weeks post-infarction (reproduced from reference 27 with permission of the author and the publisher).

that an approximately 5 dB difference in the average integrated backscatter is present between normal and acutely ischemic myocardium. The correction factor compensates primarily for the low-pass filter effect of the chest wall.

Subsequently, Barzilai et al. used the EKG gated system previously described to evaluate in dogs the effects of ischemia induced by LAD artery ligation on the amplitude of cyclic variation in backscatter [21]. By 30 minutes post-occlusion, average backscatter values were elevated as in prior observations; in addition, the normal 3.5 dB decline from end-diastole to end-systole was lost. This observation was reproduced by Glueck et al., and was found to be present as early as 10 minutes post-occlusion (Figure 6) [22]. Due to the dependence on location of cyclic variation in backscatter, assessment of ischemia by the amplitude of cyclic fluctuation would be most sensitive in apical segments, and of limited value in basilar segments.

Using the statistical measure mean amplitude/standard deviation of the amplitude (MSR), Schnittger et al. evaluated acute ischemia in 10 dogs following ligation of the LAD [24]. A 3.5 MHz phased-array transducer was used for anatomical orientation in two dimensions, and the unprocessed radio frequency backscatter signal was digitized at 20 MHz in mid-diastole along a cursor-selected M-mode line. An 8-bit transient recorder was used to sample 40 M-mode scan lines in sequence over 40 msec. Studies from a region of interest in the infarct risk area were obtained in open chest dogs, and repeated with the chest closed. The MSR was increased significantly at 30 min post-occlusion and remained elevated for the 4 hour duration of study (Figure 8). Results were unaffected by the presence of intervening chest wall [24].

Qualitative assessment of the 2D echocardiographic appearance of acute myocardial infarction in dogs indicates that increased echo amplitude may be discerned within 15 minutes of coronary ligation [8]. Parisi found that visual perception of acute infarction by 2D echocardiography was enhanced by color encoding [43]. Quantitative 2D echocardiographic studies were performed by Skorton et al. using a 2.4 MHz phased array scanner to evaluate regional mean gray level and gray level histograms at end-diastole and end-systole [45]. Seven closed-chest dogs were imaged before and 2 days after left circumflex coronary artery occlusion. The average gray level in the infarct region, located in the posterior wall of the left ventricle, was nearly twice that of control gray level. Gray level histograms (frequency of occurrence of pixels at each gray level) plotted from these same infarct regions exhibited a significant decrease in kurtosis (flattened gray level distribution). Gray level histogram distributions, but not average gray level, could distinguish normal from infarcted regions in the post-occlusion images [45]. Haendchen et al. studied regional average pixel intensity and gray level histogram distributions in 8 closed-chest dogs prior to LAD artery ligation, and repeated measurements at 1 and 3 hours post-ligation [46]. Using a 5 MHz mechanical sector scanner, end-diastolic images of the left ventricle were obtained and partitioned into epicardial and endocardial portions for separate analysis. There were no significant differences between control, 1 hour, or three hour post-ligation regional pixel intensities or gray level histogram distributions [46]. The above findings suggest that quantitative video echo amplitude changes that accompany acute infarction may require between 3 and 48 hours to manifest. McPherson et al. employed quantitative texture measures to assess acute infarction in 9 dogs with left circumflex artery occlusion [62]. Significant texture changes with infarction were present in systolic but not diastolic images. Texture parameters most reliably identified infarction when calculated perpendicular to the scan lines.

Rasmussen et al. directly accessed analog radio frequency signals at the peak of the EKG T wave, prior to video detection, for off-line computer analysis [38]. Average regional integrated backscatter ratios were calculated with reference to the specular reflection (ratio 1.0) at the posterior left ventricular endocardium. In the majority of five open and five closed chest dogs with left circumflex artery occlusion and full thickness infarction, the integrated backscatter ratio increased from control values of less than 0.85 to approximately 1.0 or more in regions of infarction within 10 minutes of occlusion. Values did not exceed 1.2 by 4 hours post-occlusion. Despite major differences in the methods used, these findings parallel the backscatter data of O'Donnell et al.; however the amount of increase in the backscatter with infarction was substantially lower.

78

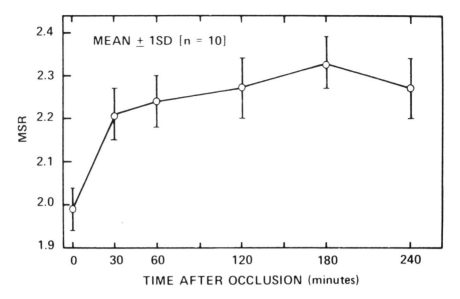

Fig. 8. In acute infarction, the statistical measure mean amplitude/standard deviation of the amplitude (MSR) increases significantly by 30 minutes after coronary occlusion (reproduced from reference 24 with permission of the author and the American Heart Association, Inc.).

Reperfusion of ischemic myocardium
In the above study by Rasmussen et al. the effect of 20 minutes of occlusion followed by reperfusion on the integrated backscatter ratio was evaluated in 2 dogs [38]. The integrated backscatter ratios were increased by 7 and 12 minutes post-occlusion, and normalized after 30 minutes of reperfusion. Glueck et al. reported the amplitude of cyclic fluctuation of the integrated backscatter at the apex in 4 dogs after LAD artery occlusion [22]. The amplitude of characteristic cyclic fluctuation was markedly reduced after 10 minutes of occlusion. Perfusion was reestablished at 10 minutes, and the amplitude of cyclic fluctuation gradually returned towards normal within 2 hours (Figure 6). The absolute value of integrated backscatter increased by approximately 2.3 dB after ten minutes of occlusion, then fell by 0.6 dB back towards normal after 2 hours of reperfusion. Following 3 hours of LAD artery occlusion in 8 dogs, Haendchen et al. found a substantial increase in 2D echocardiographic regional pixel intensity at 5 minutes of reperfusion, which persisted for an hour of observation prior to pathologic study [46]. The amount of increase in average regional pixel intensity corresponded to quantitative estimates of the extent of irreversibly injured myocardium. A parallel decrease in the skewness of regional gray level histogram distributions was also observed.

Chronic myocardial infarction
Mimbs et al. demonstrated that by 3 days post-infarction, attenuation of ultra-

sound in the myocardium increased over the control level, and was futher elevated at 6 weeeks post-infarction [27]. In other experiments with dog hearts, the attenuation increase at 4–5 or 9–11 weeks post-infarction was related to myocardial creatine kinase depletion, an independent marker of ischemic damage [33]. The index of attenuation correlated moderately well with creatine kinase depletion (r=0.80 and 0.72 respectively), implying that attenuation was sensitive to the quantitative extent of regional necrosis post-infarction.

Theoretical considerations of connective tissue density and elastic moduli have suggested that this tissue component, which is composed primarily of collagen fibers, may interact in a significant way with ultrasound [35]. Accordingly, Mimbs et al. studied in vitro the attenuation and collagen content in 110 regions from 18 dog hearts at 2, 4, and 6 weeks following LAD artery occlusion [32]. There was a linear correlation between the collagen content, as estimated by hydroxyproline assay, and the index of attenuation. The correlation coefficient increased (r=0.73, 0.77, and 0.90 at 2, 4, and 6 weeks respectively) with maturation of the scarring process at each successive time interval. Regional attenuation was also increased in five isolated perfused rabbit hearts studied at 5–7 weeks post-infarction. Addition of collagenase to the perfusate did not influence the regional collagen content or attenuation, although collagen degradation did occur, as evidenced by softening of the myocardium [32]. The 2.25 MHz backscatter coefficient was also evaluated 5–7 weeks post-infarction in this rabbit heart model, and was found to be increased nearly tenfold (-58.0 ± 2.4 [SE] dB in non-ischemic regions, versus -38.8 ± 2.2 dB for infarct regions). This was associated with a sixfold increase in the regional collagen content ($0.54 \pm 0.03\%$ wet weight in non-ischemic regions versus $3.58 \pm 0.42\%$ for infarct regions). Unlike the attenuation index, addition of collagenase to the perfusate did result in a decline of the backscatter coefficient towards normal levels (-45.1 ± 1.2 dB) [32]. These findings indicate that the backscatter, but not attenuation, is related to specifically intact collagen.

O'Donnell et al. further investigated in vitro the backscatter coefficient and regional collagen content at 5–6 weeks, 8–10 weeks, and 15–17 weeks after LAD artery occlusion [40]. There were from 30–36 sites evaluated for three groups of five or six dogs at each time interval after occlusion. The backscatter coefficient was increased substantially by 5–6 weeks after occlusion, particularly in the 2–3 MHz range. An additional increase in the backscatter coefficient was observed by 8–10 weeks, and by 15–17 weeks little additional change had occurred. The average hydroxyproline content of noninfarcted myocardium was 1.0 mg/g wet weight. Hydroxyproline content increased to 8.15 mg/g by 5–6 weeks, and to 10.15 mg/g by 8–10 weeks, remaining near this level at 15–17 weeks post-infarction. Quantitative increases in the backscatter coefficient were not in proportion to myocardial collagen content for the 5–6 week to 8–10 week post-infarction interval. O'Donnell et al. suggested a possible explanation for this finding by postulating that, in addition to total collagen (hydroxyproline) content, the organizational state of collagen in a developing scar may influence backscattering [40]. In the development of scar tissue, fibroblasts synthesize helical molecules of tropocollagen, which cross-link to form collagen fibrils with a characteristic periodicity of 60–70 nm. Fibrils in turn combine to form structural collagen fibers. Wavelength to particle size considerations indicate molecular and fibrillar collagen are probably too small to be efficient scatterers of ultrasound in the low frequency range, whereas larger organized collagen fibers appear to be the dominant acoustic scatterer in regions of chronic infarction.

Hoyt et al. evaluated in vitro the 2.25 MHz integrated backscatter and collagen content in postmortem human left ventricles with remote myocardial infarction [63]. Collagen content was estimated by hydroxyproline assay, and spatial details of collagen deposition were quantitated by a computer-assisted histologic analysis system. There was a significant correlation between the integrated backscatter and logarithm of hydroxyproline content of the myocardium (r=0.81). A fair correlation (r=0.51) was found between spatially localized fluctuations of the backscatter amplitude and foci of collagen deposition. In addition, increases in subendocardial backscatter amplitude were closely related to remote subendocardial infarction.

Parisi et al. noted that the color encoded echo intensity in 2D echocardiographic images of dog hearts became maximal at 6–8 weeks post-infarction, and corresponded to myocardial scar formation [43]. Shaw et al. used a 3 MHz center frequency transducer to obtain 2D echocardiograms in four patients with coronary artery disease, and 16 patients with valvular or congenital heart disease, within one week preceding death [64]. The median pixel gray level in regions of interest from end-diastolic images was assigned to one of seven levels. Postmortem examination permitted estimation of hydroxyproline content from these same regions. When regions of septal hypertrophy were excluded, there was a linear correlation between median gray level and the logarithm of collagen content (r=0.76) [64]. No subsequent 2D echocardiographic studies have been performed to evaluate average gray level, gray level histogram distributions, or image texture in either experimental or human chronic myocardial infarction.

Cardiomyopathy

Qualitative echocardiographic findings in cardiomyopathy were mentioned previously, and only limited quantitative data is available. Despite this paucity of data, noninvasive assessment of cardiomyopathy remains an area of tremendous potential clinical application for tissue characterization. In an effort to determine if ultrasonic backscatter is sensitive to cardiomyopathy, Mimbs et al. studied a rabbit model of anthracycline cardiotoxicity [65]. Using a 5 MHz center frequency focused transducer, the left ventricles of 15 rabbits were studied 10–18 weeks after administration of doxorubicin. The presence of cardiomyopathy was

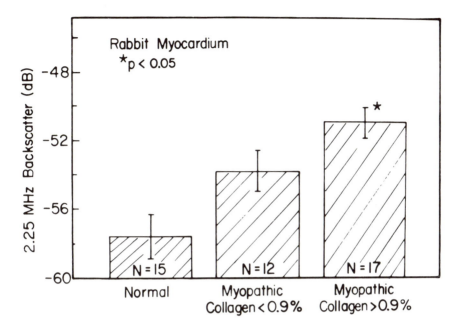

Fig. 9. In doxorubicin-treated rabbits, ultrasonic backscatter parallels the collagen content of mildly and severely myopathic left ventricle (reproduced from reference 65 with permission of the author and the publisher).

determined by regional collagen content as estimated by hydroxyproline assay. Results were arbitrarily divided into mild (collagen $< 0.9\%$ wet weight) or severe (collagen $> 0.9\%$) myopathic change. With this division, it was possible to demonstrate a trend relating collagen content to the level of integrated backscatter (Figure 9). At 2.25 MHz, severely myopathic regions exhibited an average 7 dB increase in the integrated backscatter. A possible role for the use of ultrasonic backscatter to monitor anthracycline cardiotoxicity was proposed.

Perez et al. used a 25 MHz center frequency transducer to study ultrasonic attenuation and backscatter in a Syrian hamster model of cardiomyopathy [60]. These animals spontaneously develop disease of the cardiac muscle characterized by early calcification and late fibrosis. The regional integrated backscatter as well as a slope index of attenuation were measured in vitro at 100 adjacent sites to characterize the left ventricle. Two groups of 10 hamsters each were studied at 2–3 or 5–7 months of age. Calcification and fibrosis were assessed by histologic study. Age matched normal control 2–3 month old hamsters had values for backscatter clustered around -58.07 ± 0.08 (SE) dB, whereas Syrian hamsters with predominant calcification exhibited a broad distribution of values (as high as -38 dB) with a higher average integrated backscatter of -58.87 ± 0.26 dB. In 5–7 month old Syrian hamsters, with both myocardial calcification and fibrosis, the average backscatter increased to -50.87 ± 0.22 dB with a similar wide

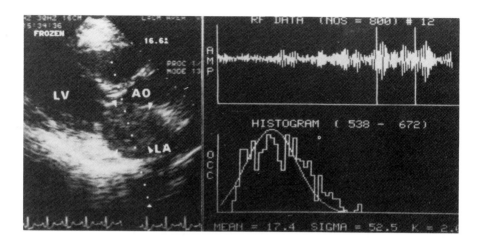

Fig. 10. Composite figure demonstrating stochastic analysis of a left atrial myxoma. Amplitude data from the region of interest in a 2D echocardiogram is acquired along an M-mode cursor (upper left, Ao = aortic root, LV = left ventricle, LA = left atrium). The upper right panel shows an unprocessed radio frequency signal, plotted as amplitude (ordinate) versus depth (abscissa). The lower right panel depicts the fit of actual data points to a random probability density function, demonstrating a correlated component of scattering from the myxomatous tissue (reproduced from reference 37 with permission of the author and the publisher).

distribution of values. Chanrasekaran et al. studied the 2D echocardiograms of patients with cardiomyopathy [66]. Ten patients each had either hypertrophic cardiomyopathy or amyloidosis. Quantitative texture measures were able to distinguish those with hypertrophic cardiomyopathy, but not amyloid infiltration, from normals.

Miscellaneous conditions

Allan et al. used color encoding of 2D echocardiograms to facilitate recognition of cardiac tumors in infants [44]. Green et al. have applied off-line digital signal analysis of radio frequency amplitude data to evaluate the composition of intra-cardiac masses in 15 patients [37]. The k value describing amplitude histograms was useful in distinguishing thrombi, tumors, and artifacts (Figure 10). In experimental myocardial contusion in dogs, Skorton et al. differentiated normal from contused myocardium by quantitative texture analysis of 2D echocardiographic images along the azimuthal (lateral) direction [47].

Summary

Information has been accumulated to indicate that abnormal myocardium can be distinguished from control normal regions by ultrasonic analysis in a variety of disease states. The specificity of such changes for the differential diagnosis of an unknown heart disease is much less clear. For example, increases of more than 5 dB in the integrated backscatter have been reported in acute and chronic infarction, cardiomyopathy, and between the normal left and right ventricles. Moreover, there exists only a limited understanding of the nature of ultrasonic interaction with normal and diseased myocardium, although muscle fibers, collagen fibers, and tissue water content all appear to have important roles. Since the relationships between the various modalities proposed for acoustic characterization of the myocardium are not fully clarified, additional data are needed to assist in determination of the approach(es) most applicable to specific categories of myocardial disease.

Present day clinical noninvasive imaging techniques are not designed to provide the type of information characterizing myocardial structure and physiologic state which has been described in this chapter. Thus, the clinical potential for addition of ultrasonic characterization of the myocardium to existing echocardiographic methods is significant. Further improvements in instrumentation and analytical techniques are expected to evolve rapidly.

References

1. Rasmussen S, Corya BC, Feigenbaum H, Knoebel SB: Detection of myocardial scar tissue by M-mode echocardiography. Circulation 1978; 57: 230–237.
2. Martin RP, Rakowski H, French J, Popp RL: Idiopathic hypertrophic subaortic stenosis viewed by wide-angle, phased-array echocardiography. Circulation 1979; 59: 1206–1217.
3. Tanaka M, Terasawa Y: Echocardiography: evaluation of the tissue character in myocardium. Japan Circ J 1979; 43: 367–376.
4. Siqueira-Filho AG, Cunha CLP, Tajik AJ, Seward JB, Schattenberg TT, Giuliani ER: M-mode and two-dimensional echocardiographic features in cardiac amyloidosis. Circulation 1981; 63: 188–196.
5. Davies J, Gibson DG, Foale R, Heer K, Spry CJF, Oakley CM, Goodwin JF: Echocardiographic features of eosinophilic endomyocardial disease. Br Heart J 1982; 48: 434–440.
6. Bhandari AK, Nanda NC, Hicks DG: Two-dimensional echocardiography of intracardiac masses: echo pattern-histopathology correlation. Ultrasound Med Biol 1982; 8: 673–680.
7. Bhandari AK, Nanda NC: Myocardial texture characterization by two-dimensional echocardiography. Am J Cardiol 1983; 51: 817–825.
8. Fraker TD Jr, Nelson AD, Arthur JA, Wilkerson RD: Altered acoustic reflectance on two-dimensional echocardiography as an early predictor of myocardial infarct size. Am J Cardiol 1984; 53: 1699–1702.
9. Garcia E, Gueret P, Bennett M, Corday E, Zwehl W, Meerbaum S, Corday S, Swan HJC, Berman D: Real time computerization of two-dimensional echocardiography. Am Heart J 1981; 101: 783–792.

10. Collins SM, Skorton DJ: Cardiac Imaging and Image Processing. New York, McGraw-Hill Book Co. 1986.
11. O'Donnell M, Bauwens D, Mimbs JW, Miller JG: Broadband integrated backscatter: an approach to spatially localized tissue characterization in vivo. Proceedings IEEE Ultrasonics Symposium 1979; pp 175–178.
12. Cohen RD, Mottley JG, Miller JG, Kurnik PB, Sobel BE: Detection of ischemic myocardium in vivo through the chest wall by quantitative ultrasonic tissue characterization. Am J Cardiol 1982; 50: 838–843.
13. Klepper JR, Brandenburger GH, Mimbs JW, Sobel BE, Miller JG: Application of phase-insensitive detection and frequency-dependent measurements to computed ultrasonic attenuation tomography. IEEE Trans Biomed Eng 1981; BME-28: 186–201.
14. Busse LJ, Miller JG, Yuhas DE, Mimbs JW, Weiss AN, Sobel BE: Phase cancellation effects: a source of attenuation artifact eliminated by a CdS acoustoelectric receiver. In: White D (ed) *Ultrasound in Medicine,* New York, Plenum Press 1977; vol. 3, pp 1519–1535.
15. Entrekin R, Melton HE: Real-time speckle reduction in B-mode images. Proceedings IEEE Ultrasonics Symposium 1979; pp 169–178.
16. Chapelon JY, Cathignol D, Fourcade C: Improved ultrasonic sensitivity using pseudo-random binary-code phase-modulated signals. Ultrasonic Imaging 1979; 1: 255–264.
17. Skorton DJ, Collins SM, Woskoff SD, Bean JA, Melton HE Jr: Range- and azimuth-dependent variability of image texture in two-dimensional echocardiograms. Circulation 1983; 68: 834–840.
18. Melton HE Jr, Skorton DJ: Rational gain compensation for attenuation in cardiac ultrasonography. Ultrasonic Imaging 1983; 5: 214–228.
19. O'Donnell M: Quantitative volume backscatter imaging. IEEE Trans Sonics Ultrasonics 1983; SU-30: 26–36.
20. Madaras EI, Barzilai B, Perez JE, Sobel BE, Miller JG: Changes in myocardial backscatter throughout the cardiac cycle. Ultrasonic Imaging 1983; 5: 229–239.
21. Barzilai B, Madaras EI, Sobel BE, Miller JG, Perez JE: Effects of myocardial contraction on ultrasonic backscatter before and after ischemia. Am J Physiol 1984; 247: H478–H483.
22. Glueck RM, Mottley JG, Miller JG, Sobel BE, Perez JE: Effects of coronary artery occlusion and reperfusion on cardiac cycle-dependent variation of myocardial ultrasonic backscatter. Circ Res 1985; 56: 683–689.
23. Gramiak R, Waag RC, Schenk EA, Lee PPK, Thomson K, Macintosh P: Ultrasonic detection of myocardial infarction by amplitude analysis. Radiology 1979; 130: 713–720.
24. Schnittger I, Vieli A, Heiserman JE, Director BA, Billingham ME, Ellis SG, Kernoff RS, Takamoto T, Popp RL: Ultrasonic tissue characterization: detection of acute myocardial ischemia in dogs. Circulation 1985; 72: 193–199.
25. Hoyt RH, Skorton DJ, Collins SM, Melton HE Jr: Ultrasonic backscatter and collagen in normal ventricular myocardium. Circulation 1984; 69: 775–782.
26. Mimbs JW, Bauwens D, Cohen RD, O'Donnell M, Miller JG, Sobel BE: Effects of myocardial ischemia on quantitative ultrasonic backscatter and identification of responsible determinants. Circ Res 1981; 49: 89–96.
27. Mimbs JW, O'Donnell M, Miller JG, Sobel BE: Changes in ultrasonic attenuation indicative of early myocardial ischemic injury. Am J Physiol 1979; 236: H340–H344.
28. Shung KK, Reid JM: Ultrasonic scattering from tissues. Proceedings IEEE Ultrasonics Symposium 1977; pp 230–233.
29. Namery J, Lele PP: Ultrasonic detection of myocardial infarction in dog. Proceedings IEEE Ultrasonics Symposium 1972; pp 491–494.
30. Gregg EC, Palagallo GL: Acoustic impedance of tissue. Invest Radiol 1969; 4: 357–363.
31. Chivers RC: Tissue characterization. Ultrasound Med Biol 1981; 7: 1–20.
32. Mimbs JW, O'Donnell M, Bauwens D, Miller JG, Sobel BE: The dependence of ultrasonic attenuation and backscatter on collagen content in dog and rabbit hearts. Circ Res 1980; 47: 49–58.

33. Mimbs JW, Yuhas DE, Miller JG, Weiss AN, Sobel BE: Detection of myocardial infarction in vitro based on altered attenuation of ultrasound. Circ Res 1977; 41: 192–198.
34. Nicholas D, Hill CR, Nassiri DK: Evaluation of backscattering coefficients for excised human tissues: principles and techniques. Ultrasound Med Biol 1982; 8: 7–15.
35. Fields S, Dunn F: Correlation of echographic visualizability of tissue with biological composition and physiological state. J Acoust Soc Am 1973; 54: 809–812.
36. Sigelmann RA, Reid JM: Analysis and measurement of ultrasound backscattering from an ensemble of scatterers excited by sine-wave bursts. J Acoust Soc Am 1972; 53: 1351–1355.
37. Green SE, Joynt LF, Fitzgerald PJ, Rubenson DS, Popp RL: In vivo ultrasonic tissue characterization of human intracardiac masses. Am J Cardiol 1983; 51: 231–236.
38. Rasmussen S, Lovelace DE, Knoebel SB, Ransburg R, Corya BC: Echocardiographic detection of ischemic and infarcted myocardium. J Am Coll Cardiol 1984; 3: 733–743.
39. Chivers RC: The scattering of ultrasound by human tissues – some theoretical models. Ultrasound Med Biol 1977; 3: 1–13.
40. O'Donnell M, Mimbs JW, Miller JG: Relationship between collagen and ultrasonic backscatter in myocardial tissue. J Acoust Soc Am 1981; 62: 580–588.
41. Fitzgerald PJ, Joynt LF, Green SE, Popp RL: Computerized echocardiographic tissue characterization. In: Computers in Cardiology. Long Beach, CA, IEEE Computer Society, 1981; pp 395–398.
42. Logan-Sinclair R, Wong CM, Gibson DG: Clinical application of amplitude processing of echocardiographic images. Br Heart J 1981; 45: 621–627.
43. Parisi AF, Nieminen M, O'Boyle JE, Moynihan PF, Khuri SF, Kloner RA, Folland ED, Schoen FJ: Enhanced detection of the evolution of tissue changes after acute myocardial infarction using color-encoded two-dimentsional echocardiography. Circulation 1982; 66: 764–770.
44. Allan LD, Joseph MC, Tynan M: Clinical value of echocardiographic colour image processing in two cases of primary cardiac tumour. Br Heart J 1983; 49: 154–156.
45. Skorton DJ, Melton HE Jr, Pandian NG, Nichols J, Koyanagi S, Marcus ML, Collins SM, Kerber RE: Detection of acute myocardial infarction in closed-chest dogs by analysis of regional two-dimensional echocardiographic gray-level distributions. Circ Res 1983; 52: 36–44.
46. Haendchen RV, Ong K, Fishbein MC, Zwehl W, Meerbaum S, Corday E: Early differentiation of infarcted and noninfarcted reperfused myocardium in dogs by quantitative analysis of regional myocardial echo amplitudes. Circ Res 1985; 57: 718–728.
47. Skorton DJ, Collins SM, Nichols J, Pandian NG, Bean JA, Kerber RE: Quantitative texture analysis in two-dimensional echocardiography: application to the diagnosis of experimental myocardial contusion. Circulation 1983; 68: 217–223.
48. Johnston RL, Goss SA, Maynard V, Brady JK, Frizzell LA, O'Brien WD Jr, Dunn F: Elements of tissue characterization, Part I. Ultrasonic propagation properties. In: Linzer M (ed) Ultrasonic tissue characterization II. Washington DC, US Government Printing Office, US Dept of Commerce, Nat Bur Stand, Spec Publ 1979; 525: 19–27.
49. O'Donnell M, Mimbs JW, Sobel BE, Miller JG: Ultrasonic attenuation in normal and ischemic myocardium. In: Linzer M (ed) Ultrasonic tissue characterization II. Washington DC, US Government Printing Office, US Dept of Commerce, Nat Bur Stand, Spec Publ 1979; 525: 63–71.
50. Mottley JG, Miller JG: Anisotropy of ultrasonic attenuation in canine heart and liver. Ultrasonic Imaging 1982; 4: 180 (abstract).
51. Nassiri D, Nicholas D, Hill CR: Scattering and attenuation in anisotropic human tissue. Proc 3rd Euro Congress for Ultrasound in Medicine 1978; pp 381 (abstract).
52. Caspari PG, Newcomb M, Gibson K, Harris P: Collagen in the normal and hypertrophied human ventricle. Cardiovasc Res 1977; 11: 554–558.
53. Buccino RA, Harris E, Spann JF Jr, Sonnenblick EH: Response of myocardial connective tissue to development of experimental hypertrophy. Am J Physiol 1969; 216: 425–428.
54. Hoyt R, Melton HE Jr, Skorton DJ: Regional variation in ultrasonic backscatter: in vitro studies

of canine myocardium. Ultrasound Med Biol 1982; 8(suppl 1): 81 (abstract).

55. Baello EB, McPherson DD, Conyers DJ, Collins SM, Skorton DJ: Acoustic properties of the normal dog heart: comparison of backscatter from all chambers. J Am Coll Cardiol 1986; (in press).

56. Oken DE, Boucek RJ: Quantitation of collagen in human myocardium. Circ Res 1957; 5: 357–361.

57. Wickline SA, Thomas LJ III, Miller JG, Sobel BE, Perez JE: The dependence of myocardial ultrasonic integrated backscatter on contractile performance. Circulation 1985; 72: 183–192.

58. Olshansky B, Collins SM, Skorton DJ, Prasad NV: Variation of left ventricular myocardial gray level on two-dimensional echocardiograms as a result of cardiac contraction. Circulation 1984; 70: 972–977.

59. Collins SM, Skorton DJ, Prasad NV, Olshansky B, Bean JA: Quantitative echocardiographic image texture: normal contraction-related variability. IEEE Trans Medical Imaging 1985; MI-4: 185–192.

60. Perez JE, Barzilai B, Madaras EI, Glueck RM, Saffitz JE, Johnston P, Miller JG, Sobel BE: Applicability of ultrasonic tissue characterization for longitudinal assessment and differentiation of calcification and fibrosis in cardiomyopathy. J Am Coll Cardiol 1984; 4: 88–95.

61. Dines KA, Weyman AE, Franklin TD Jr, Cuddeback JK, Sanghvi NT, Avery KS, Baird AI, Fry FJ: Quantitation of changes in myocardial fiber bundle spacing with acute infarction, using pulse-echo ultrasound signals. Circulation 1981; 60(suppl II): 17 (abstract).

62. McPherson DD, Aylward PE, Knosp BM, Eltoft DA, Bean JA, Kieso RA, Kerber RE, Collins SM, Skorton DJ: Ultrasound characterization of acute myocardial ischemia by polar texture analysis. Circulation 1984; 70(suppl II): 396 (abstract).

63. Hoyt RH, Collins SM, Skorton DJ, Ericksen EE, Conyers D: Assessment of fibrosis in infarcted human hearts by analysis of ultrasonic backscatter. Circulation 1985; 71: 740–744.

64. Shaw TRD, Logan-Sinclair RB, Surin C, McAnulty RJ, Heard B, Laurent GJ, Gibson DG: Relation between regional echo intensity and myocardial connective tissue in chronic left ventricular disease. Br Heart J 1984; 51: 46–53.

65. Mimbs JW, O'Donnell M, Miller JG, Sobel BE: Detection of cardiomyopathic changes induced by doxorubicin based on quantitative analysis of ultrasonic backscatter. Am J Cardiol 1981; 47: 1056–1060.

66. Chandrasekaran K, Aylward PE, Knosp BM, Collins SM, Bean JA, Seward JB, Tajik AJ, Skorton DJ: Quantitative echocardiographic texture analysis can identify cardiomyopathy in humans. Circulation 1985; 72(suppl III): 207 (abstract).

7. Clinical approaches to echocardiographic tissue characterisation

D.G. GIBSON and R.B. LOGAN SINCLAIR
Brompton Hospital, London, UK

Ultrasonic tissue characterisation aims at gaining information about the physical properties of structures under examination rather than simply registering their position and motion. This additional information comes from determining characteristics of echoes beyond those related to the time at which they return to the transducer, in order to gain an idea as to how the ultrasound has been modified during its passage through the tissues. A number of such characteristics have been used, including those of individual echoes such as amplitude, phase, or frequency content, or those involving a statistical analysis of the distribution of some property over the image, a process referred to as texture analysis. Tissue characterisation thus depends to a much greater extent than simple image generation on quantification of ultrasound. In addition, if it is to be anything other than an empirical endeavour, the physical properties of the tissues, the nature of their interaction with ultrasound and the transfer function of the system used to generate and record the ultrasound must all be characterised. As will be seen, each of these stages give rise to conceptual and practical problems.

In order to investigate this approach to tissue characterisation, we chose to quantify what appeared to be the simplest property of the returning ultrasound, namely its amplitude. Yet, before any abnormality of amplitude can be directly related to the properties of a target within the heart, a number of extraneous factors must be identified and allowed for. These include the gain and depth compensation of the echocardiograph, the frequency composition of the ultrasound leaving the transducer and its corresponding sensitivity used as a receiver, the orientation of the target with respect to the ultrasound beam, the effect of any intervening structures and the basic nature of its interaction with tissue. Unfortunately, absolute standardisation of all these factors cannot at present be achieved in the experimental, still less in the clinical setting.

In view of these difficulties, we have used simplified solutions, knowing that the results will be no more than semiquantitative. This approach could only be justified if the differences between normal and abnormal tissues were very large, an assumption that appears to have been borne out in practice. The heart has

J. Roelandt (editor), Digital Techniques in Echocardiography. ISBN 0-89838-861-9.

proved a much easier organ to study in this way than intraabdominal viscera such as the liver. Its structure is predictable, consisting of myocardium no more than 2 cm thick surrounding blood filled cavities. Posterior to the left ventricular wall is the parietal pericardium formed of dense fibrous tissue, with a uniform composition of 50–60% collagen [1] which reflects ultrasound very intensely. We have taken advantage of these factors and have standardised the overall gain of the echocardiograph by increasing it until the posterior pericardial echo is just displayed as a continuous line at the maximum grey scale level. This procedure allows for the effects of chest wall, path length and frequency-dependent attenuation. Depth compensation settings must also be standardised; its complete elimination seriously impairs overall image quality, so we have employed an arbitrary but practical solution of a linear relation between the posterior pericardium and anterior chest wall, which again is set just to the highest level of grey scale. If image generation were due to specular reflection, echo amplitude would depend critically on the orientation of the target to the ultrasound beam, so that structures would be detected only when they were perpendicular to it. Consideration of the apical views demonstrates that this cannot be the case; all four cardiac chambers are demonstrated although no structure other than the AV valve cusps during systole are perpendicular to the beam. This relative independence of amplitude on orientation has been confirmed in more formal studies [1]. It seems clear that myocardial echoes of clinical interest arise by backscattering, demonstrating their origin from targets that are small compared with the wavelength of ultrasound used. The physical basis of back scattering is very complex, but when this process is involved, reflected amplitude is very much less sensitive to direction that for specular reflection. Quantification of the extent of absorbtion of ultrasound by proximal tissues is not easy to perform. Though desirable, it is not essential in the setting of the anatomical structure of the heart, since it is quite possible to establish relatively narrow normal ranges for myocardium in well defined regions such as septum, papillary muscle, or posterior wall in each cut, and to alter the relative positions of structures by imaging from the different windows.

A major problem in the extraction of quantitative information has arisen directly from current ideas on the design of equipment for clinical use. It would appear that manufacturers are more concerned with the subjective, or even the aesthetic qualities of the image, at the expense of quantitation, so that facilities for acoustic and electrical calibration are not provided. Indeed, considerable effort appears to have been devoted to the development of post-processing manipulations which cause minor changes in the appearance of the image by altering grey scale, though their use has not been shown to have any diagnostic significance. This state of affairs has arisen because commercially available instruments are designed to demonstrate interfaces rather than absolute amplitude levels within tissues. The question of calibration of echocardiographic equipment is clearly crucial to any attempt at tissue characterisation but has been little addressed. A microprocessor controlled system has thus been developed, capable of single and multiple burst linear transmission and data acquisition, at the same time maintaining maximum machine variable independence. It depends on injecting signals of known characteristics into the transducer from a second crystal. The test rig consists of a cylindrical tank with the scanner transducer mounted at its top. An NPL calibrated 4 mm membrane hydrophone is mounted 10 mm below it to measure test signal characteristics. Precise control of amplitude, frequency, timing, and wave shape is available, allowing the scanner to be calibrated in absolute units of acoustic pressure. A second hydrophone, mounted 60 mm below the transducer allows the characteristics of the transmitted pulses to be determined.

Echo amplitude is traditionally displayed a grey scale, but this is not entirely satisfactory, since values are greatly affected by the exact settings of the instruments, while the dynamic range of currently available copy is not always adequate to convey the information satisfactorily. In addition, perceived levels of grey scale depend on the distribution of absolute values across the image, so that ambiguities may develop, giving rise to effects such as that described by Craik and O'Brien. For these reasons, a system of colour and amplitude encoding seemed preferable, colour substitution alone causing a reduction in image quality [1]. This has proved an excellent system for giving an overall impression of amplitude values. The equipment runs in real time, and is routinely used for selecting appropriate gain settings at the time when the images are recorded. In order to quantify regional echo levels, an area of interest of 200–300 pixels is selected on a video stop frame, and a histogram of their intensities constructed. Overall pixel intensity is expressed as the median level [2], Figure 1. The standard deviation of the reproducibility between duplicate determinations made in this way is 0.41 grey scale unit. Comparison between automatic and manual pixel counting showed the standard deviation of the difference between the two determinations to be 0.58 unit. Further information as to the kurtosis is also potentially available [3], subject to limitation by the relatively small number of pixels counted. Echo intensity may also vary during the cardiac cycle [4], so that all measurements are performed on end-diastolic images. This variation of intensity during the cardiac cycle can be demonstrated on a colour M-mode display, so that changes across the wall as well as those between systole and diastole can be localised and measured. It is possible that they may reflect corresponding alterations in myocardial stiffness as tension changes throughout the cardiac cycle.

Several lines of evidence have suggested that connective tissue may be an important determinant of the intensity of 'structural' echoes as distinct from those arising from interfaces between organs. The stiffness of collagen is very much greater than that of any tissue other than bone, and in breast, reflectivity is closely related to fibrosis [5]. In experimental animals after experimental myocardial infarction, or with daunorubicin induced cardiotoxicity [6, 7], considerable increases in the intensity of integrated backscattering can be detected. In man, an

90

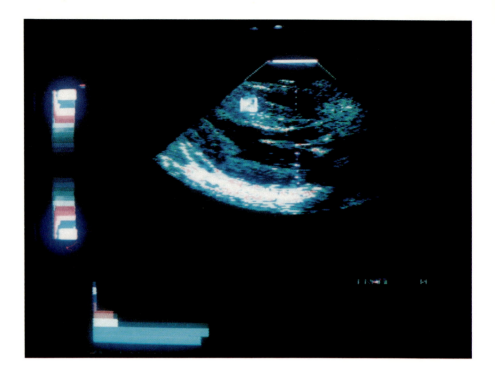

Fig. 1. Left ventricular hypertrophy. Long axis parasternal view, showing increased septal and posterior wall thickness. The colour sequence used to encode echo intensity is shown on the upper left. In this patient, myocardial echo intensity, displayed as predominately green, is normal. An area of interest has been positioned over the septum, and a histogram of pixel intensity is shown horizontally in the lower part of the display.

increase in the intensity of septal echoes has been documented by M-mode echocardiography in patients with old infarction [8], and more recently, fibrosis has been identified as the cause of high intensity echoes in the septum on 2D displays [9]. Our own experience with patients with coronary artery disease or eosinophilic heart disease is similar [10, 11].

In order to examine any relation between fibrosis and echo amplitude in greater detail, echocardiograms recorded within one week of death in 19 patients were compared with autopsy material [2]. Myocardium was taken from the free wall of the left ventricle, the septum, and the papillary muscles and its connective tissue content assessed histologically in terms of fibrosis, and biochemically, as hydroxyproline. Myocardial echo intensity was found to correlate in a linear manner with log collagen concentration. The calibration curve of the septum differed from that of the posterior wall in demonstrating consistently higher levels of echo intensity at any given collagen concentration. However, within these two regions, values from infants were identical to those of adults, demonstrating the validity of the method of calibrating the gain of the echocardiograph in allowing for changes in path length and frequency-dependent attenuation. Agreement between echo intensity and histological estimates of fibrosis was poor, but histology also correlated poorly with biochemical determinations. In retrospect, it seems likely that orthodox histology is subject to sampling errors since fibrosis is not uniformly distributed. In addition, the volume sampled for a histological section is very much less than that used for a biochemical determination, itself less than that effectively sampled for an ultrasound measurement. The solution appears to be a substantial increase in the number of histological sections studied, using an automatic method based on pixel counting. Nevertheless, these findings underline the importance of not relying on a single 'gold standard' in such studies. They stress difficulties in quantifying the extent of a tissue abnormality even when it is apparently so well defined as 'fibrosis'. Such difficulties are likely to become more prominent as efforts at echocardiographic tissue characterisation proceed.

The ability to detect the presence and distribution of fibrous tissue within the myocardium of the ventricles gives information which is frequently of clinical interest and sometimes of therapeutic significance. In patients with coronary artery disease, myocardial scar can be localised. In those in whom a diagnosis of papillary muscle dysfunction has been made on the basis of a soft apical pan-systolic murmur, areas of increased echo intensity within the papillary muscles can regularly be identified, our histological study suggesting that this can be done with considerable reliability at this site. Subendocardial fibrosis may also be very prominent. In patients with chronic rheumatic mitral valve disease, the extent and severity of subvalvular involvement can be identified more precisely than with grey scale imaging. Examination of the hypertrophied left ventricle has proved of interest. When hypertrophy is physiological, as occurs in athletes, myocardial echo intensity is normal. However, when hypertrophy is secondary to valve disease or hypertension, then echo intensity is sometimes increased [11]. This is most striking in children with left ventricular outflow tract obstruction. Its exact basis is not clear. Its presence does not correlate with coronary artery disease, but is strongly associated both with the appearance of repolarisation changes on the ECG, the so-called 'strain' pattern, and also with the characteristic series of diastolic abnormalities demonstrable by M-mode echocardiography, including prolongation of isovolumic relaxation time, reduced rate of dimension increase and wall thinning, and cavity shape changes before mitral valve opening [12]. Septal echo amplitude in patients with hypertrophic cardiomyopathy is increased no more than in patients with secondary left ventricular hypertrophy of comparable degree; we have found no evidence that the so-called 'ground glass' appearance described in grey scale images has as its basis any specific increase in amplitude [13]. In certain diseases, the pattern of distribution of increased echo amplitude may be very specific. In eosinophilic heart disease, it is found most commonly in the region of the posterior cusp of the mitral valve, and also in the inner at the bases of the papillary muscles, apparently spreading from the endo-towards the epicardium, and at the apex of the right ventricle, where the modera-

92

tor band is often involved [10]. Almost identical appearances are seen in EMF as it occurs in South India, providing further evidence of a basic similarity between the two conditions [11]. In endocardial fibroelastosis, a bright ring representing increased echo amplitude is apparent just below the endocardium, allowing the condition to be differentiated from dilated cardiomyopathy, where, as in adults, myocardial echo intensity is usually normal. As might be expected, calcification also gives rise to echoes of considerable magnitude. Though this can be detected in valve cusps, knowledge of its presence seldom changes the diagnosis or clinical management. However, it has proved possible to use the method to study the condition that occurs commonly in the elderly, so called mitral ring calcification. This can be seen to involve the base of the posterior cusp and not the mitral ring, which in any case is an insubstantial structure, the anterior cusp of the mitral valve, the aortic valve cusps, the central fibrous body and the upper part of the muscular septum where its presence may compromise the conducting system.

A second condition that might potentially be recognised from quantitative estimates of echo amplitude is myocardial inflammation. Myocarditis is a condition whose presence is frequently invoked to explain ventricular disease of apparently rapid onset, but the diagnosis is seldom unequivocally documented. Endomyocardial biopsy may show evidence of inflammation, but since only a small area of myocardium is examined, the possibility of sampling errors is appreciable. In addition, there is no general agreement as to criteria for the diagnosis of chronic inflammation [14]. In only a very small number of cases has a causative organism been recovered from the myocardium. A related and much better defined condition is myocardial rejection. It is a major concern after cardiac transplantation, and right ventricular biopsy is the standard method by which the diagnosis is made. In order to investigate the possibility that increased myocardial echo amplitude might occur with acute rejection, an animal model consisting of a heterotopic dog heart has been used. In the absence of immunosuppression, histological features of acute rejection with complete loss of function develop over a period of 6–8 days. Echocardiographic changes are already apparent by the second day after transplant, and these progress, so that by 5–8 days, there is a striking increase in echo amplitude, often of 3 or more grey scale levels (20 dB) [14]. The increase is not uniformly distributed, being much more marked in the septum than in the posterior wall of the left ventricle. The transplanted heart was biopsied, and correlation between echo level and the histological grade of rejection was demonstrated. Echo amplitude was shown to increase at approximately the time of cellular infilatration. It followed isolated myocardial oedema, but clearly preceded myocyte necrosis. These findings have been confirmed in the clinical setting, where biopsy proced episodes of acute rejection are accompanied by a striking increase in echo amplitude (Figure 2) (unpublished observations). It is of interest that these changes in the structure of the myocardium are accompanied by reproducible changes in diastolic function which can be detected by the M-mode technique, indicating that echocardiogra-

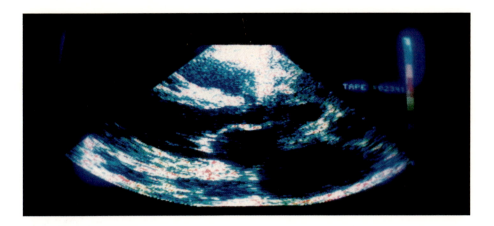

Fig. 2. Acute rejection in man. Parasternal long axis view. There is a considerable increase in myocardial echo intensity involving the posterior wall and the interventricular septum. A small pericardial effusion is also present. Myocardial thickness and calculated mass were normal. (Reproduced by permission of Dr K. Dawkins.)

phy may have a significant role to play in the non-invasive follow-up of these patients.

Observations of echo amplitude in spontaneously occurring myocarditis have been few. In the early stage of eosinophilic heart disease, a generalised increase may be present throughout the myocardium, falling later in the disease, except in specific areas. This, in association with biopsy correlations, suggests that inflammation as well as fibrosis is detected in the early stage, with the former, but not the latter regressing (Figures 3 and 4). We also seen similar increases in patients with infective endocarditis involving the left ventricular myocardium. In all of 4 with acute rheumatic fever there was an increase in echo amplitude in the sub-epirather than the sub-endocardial region.

These studies demonstrate some of the difficulties and possibilities of a very simple method of tissue characterisation, based on quantification of echo amplitude. Clearly, many further approaches are possible, either singly or in combination, though it seems likely that increased complexity and absolute quantification will be obtained only at the expense of clinical versatility. Problems are likely to arise with patients in whom high quality records cannot be obtained, and with limited reproducibility even in those in whom signal to noise ratio is high. Precise determination of the tissue abnormalities themselves may well present difficulties, obvious examples occurring should echocardiography be used to detect such relatively ill-defined entities as 'ischaemia' or 'infarct size'. On the other hand, the potential advantages of gaining more information about the physical properties of myocardium are considerable, particularly in the field of cardiomyopathy. Angiography, nuclear or contrast, or conventional echocardiography

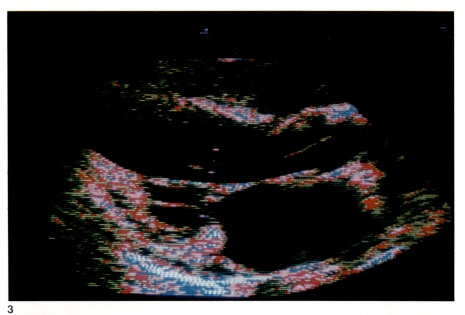

3

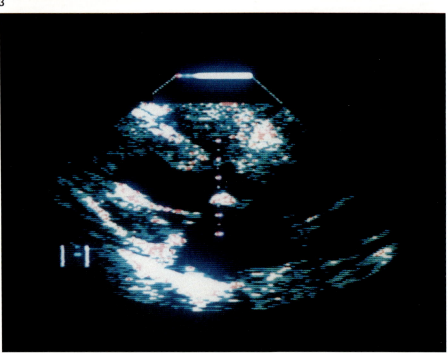

4

Fig. 3. Eosinophilic Heart Disease. Long axis parasternal view recorded in the acute stage of the illness at a time when endomyocardial biopsy showed inflammatory changes as well as fibrosis. There is a considerable increase in myocardial echo amplitude involving the septum, the posterior wall and the papillary muscles.

Fig. 4. Eosinophilic Heart Disease. Long axis parasternal view from the same patient as in figure 3, recorded 2 years later. There has been a reduction in echo amplitude in much of the posterior wall, so that now the abnormalities are concentrated in the subepicardial region, at the base of the papillary muscles, and in the region of the posterior cusp of the mitral valve.

have been used to study the interface between blood and myocardium, and it is from the position and motion of this interface that virtually all clinical information about myocardial function is derived. This state of affairs is now changing. The development of Doppler flow mapping has made it possible to document the motion of blood within the cavity, while echocardiographic tissue characterisation will take its place with other emerging technology such as NMR imaging in making accessible information about the myocardium itself.

References

1. Logan-Sinclair RB, Wong CM, Gibson DG: Clinical application of amplitude processing of echocardiographic images. Br Heart J 1981; 45: 621–627.
2. Shaw TRD, Logan-Sinclair RB, Surin C, McAnulty RJ, Heard B, Laurent GJ, Gibson DG: Relation between regional echo intensity and myocardial connective tissue in chronic left ventricular disease. Br Heart J 1984; 51: 46–53.
3. Skorton DJ, Melton Jr HE, Pandian NG, Nichols J, Koyanagi S, Marcus ML, Collins SM, Kerber RE: Detection of acute myocardial infarction in closed-chest dogs by analysis of regional two-dimensional echocardiographic gray-scale levels. Circ Res 1983; 52: 36–44.
4. Wickline SA, Thomas III LJ, Miller JG, Sobel BE, Perez JE: The dependence of myocardial ultrasonic integrated backscatter on contractile performance. Circulation 1985; 72: 183–192.
5. Fields S, Dunn F: Correlation of echocardiographic visibility of tissue with biological composition and physiological state. J Acoust Soc Am 1973; 54: 809–812.
6. Mimbs JW, Yuhas DE, Miller JG, Weiss AN, Sobel BE: Detection of myocardial infarction in vitro based on altered attenuation of ultrasound. Circ Res 1977; 41: 192–198.
7. Mimbs JW, O'Donnell M, Miller JG, Sobel BE: Detection of cardiomyopathic changes induced by doxorubicin based on quantitative analysis of ultrasonic backscatter. Am J Cardiol 1981; 47: 1056–1060.
8. Rasmussen S, Corya BC, Feigenbaum H, Knoebel SB: Detection of myocardial scar tissue by M-mode echocardiography. Circulation 1978; 57: 230–237.
9. Tanaka M, Terasawa H: Echocardiography: evaluation of tissue character in myocardium. Jpn Heart J 1979; 43: 367–376.
10. Davies J, Gibson DG, Foale R, Heer K, Spry CJF, Oakley CM, Goodwin JF: Echocardiographic features of eosinophilic endomyocardial disease. Br Heart J 1982; 48: 434–440.
11. Vijayaraghavan G, Davies J, Sandavan S, Spry C, Gibson DG, Goodwin JF: Two-D echocardiographic diagnosis of endocardial fibrosis: abnormalities of regional intensity. Circulation 1982; 66: II–122.

12. Shapiro LM, Moore RB, Logan-Sinclair RB, Gibson DG: Relation of regional echo amplitude to left ventricular function and the electrocardiogram in left ventricular hypertrophy. Br Heart J 1984; 52: 99–105.

13. Martin RP, Rakowski H, French J, Popp RL: Idiopathic hypertrophic subaortic stenosis viewed by wide-angle phased array echocardiography. Circulation 1979; 59: 1206–1217.

14. Billingham ME, Mason JW: Endomyocardial biopsy diagnosis of myocarditis and changes following immunosuppressive therapy. Viral Heart Disease. Ed. Bolte H-D. Springer Verlag, Berlin. 1984; pp 200–210.

Part Three: Left Ventricular Function

8. Automatic Contour Finding and Digital Subtraction Technique in 2-Dimensional Echocardiography

Eberhard GRUBE, Harald BECHER and Bernd BACKS
Medizinische Universitätsklinik Bonn, FRG

Left ventricular endocardium is the most important cardiac structure to calculate left ventricular function parameters such as volumes, ejection fraction and wall motion. The accurate and reproducible detection of endocardium remains the most crucial and the most important step in the quantitative analysis of 2-D echocardiograms [1–8].

Therefore the descriptive and quantitative analysis of left ventricular function is the most widely used form of interpretation of this important diagnostic screening procedure [9, 10]. The quantitative and objective analysis of 2-D echocardiographic data, however, is desirable and even mandatory for the documentation of follow-up studies and interventional procedures such as coronary lysis therapy or coronary angioplasty [11].

The inaccurate and incomplete delineation of the endocardial borders in 2-D echocardiograms, particularly with minor qualities, resulted in large interobserver variabilities and limited reproducibility of these data [12]. Automated edge detection, entered in the computer memory, therefore, should simplify and expedite the process of reproducible border detection and should allow to calculate a variety of structural and functional indices of cardiac performance [13–20]. The interobserver variability in the quantitative analysis of LV-function is largely due to the limitations for precise measurements:

- the widely used and recommended leading edge measurements are unprecise because of the lack of definite border delineation.
- the gain dependence of the echo reflection properties and
- in apical projections endocardium is only weakly reflected because of its parallel position to the interrogating sound beam.

In general, automatic contour finding algorithm should be accurate, reliable, fast and reproducible; it should also work in noisy images, should be independent of preset grey levels in the ultrasound instrument, should detect and eliminate accurately intra- and extracavitary artefacts, close endocardial gaps and adequately smooth the endocardial strings. Most importantly, however, the auto-

J. Roelandt (editor), Digital Techniques in Echocardiography. ISBN 0-89838-861-9.

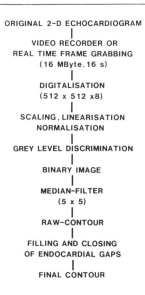

Fig. 1. Flow diagram of semi-automatic contour finding.

matically generated contour should correspond to the 'a priori' information of the left ventricle.

In general, automatic contour generation consists of the following steps [14]:
– image pre-processing in order to increase signal to noise ratio,
– application of the edge detection algorithm,
– identification and classification of endocardial strings,
– filling of endocardial gaps and finally
– elimination of artefacts and
– smoothing of endocardial raw contours.

In order to prove the accuracy and the reproducibility of automatic contour finding algorithms, we performed in-vitro experiments with formalin fixed animal hearts [18]. We examined 29 excised animal hearts which were fixed in 10% formalin solution for 7 days; out of these 29 hearts we cut 42 short axis slices with a maximal thickness of 1 cm. These short axis slices were suspended in distilled water and examined echo-cardiographically by a 3.5 mHz ultrasound probe with a phased array system. The endocardial contour and the enclosed ventricular cavity area were identified manually (via an X-Y tablet), semiautomatically and automatically. The results were then compared with the 'true areas' generated and measured by photographic prints.

A flow scheme of the semi-automatic contour generation is shown in Figure 1. Semi-automatic contour finding consists mostly of interactive steps, performed by the observer. The original 2-D echocardiogram is digitized preferably with a

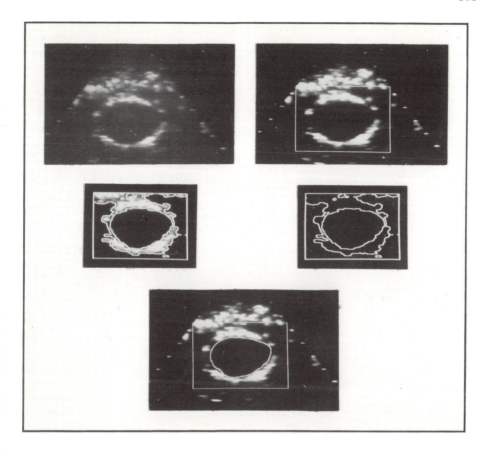

Fig. 2. In the upper part of the figure the original (left) and enhanced (right) short axis echocardiogram with the region of interest is shown; the weak echos are enhanced and the background noise is eliminated. In the middle part the semi-automatically generated contour with and without echocardiogram is displayed. In the lower part the manually drawn endocardial contour in the short axis slice is demonstrated.

$512 \times 512 \times 8$ bit grey level matrix. The pre-processing of the echocardiogram consists of scaling, linearisation and normalisation of grey levels in order to increase the definition of weak echoes and suppress high and intense echoes. These interactive steps should increase the signal to noise ratio, particularly in poor quality echocardiograms. Following image pre-processing the grey levels are discriminated and the original grey level image is converted into a binary image only containing black and white information. The grey level threshold is calculated on the basis of average grey levels in the left ventricular cavity. The program for the definition of the endocardial contour is based on the detection of the black and white borders between the left ventricular cavity and the endocardium [16].

The endocardial string is followed automatically and the edges are marked by

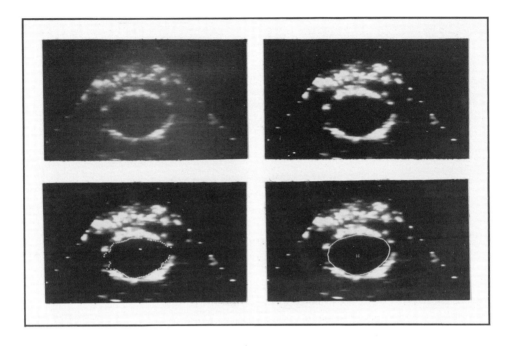

Fig. 3. In this figure the different steps of automatic contour generation are displayed: original and interactively enhanced echocardiogram in the upper part and the endocardial 'raw'- and final contours are shown.

colored contour points which are stored in the computer memory as X-Y coordinates; all points then represent the continuous endocardial border. An example of a semi-automatically generated contour is shown in Figure 2. On this graph the original echocardiogram, the pre-processed image and the semi-automatically generated contour with and without underlying echocardiograms are shown. For comparison the manually drawn contour is depicted in the lower part of this figure.

The endocardial border generated automatically by the edge detection algorithm is demonstrated in Figure 3. In this figure one can see the original and enhanced echocardiographic images as well as the automatically generated raw and final contours.

Out of 42 2-D echocardiographic images we were able to derive manually drawn contours in all 42 images. In 33 slices we were able to generate the endocardial border semi-automatically and in 30 slices automatically. If endocardial gaps were greater than 30% of the total left ventricular circumference, we considered these gaps too large in order to achieve reproducible and reliable results and classified these images as unable for automatic contour generation.

We compared the semi-automatically, automatically and manually derived contours with 'true contours' and were able to prove that these contours correl-

AUTOMATIC CONTOUR FINDING

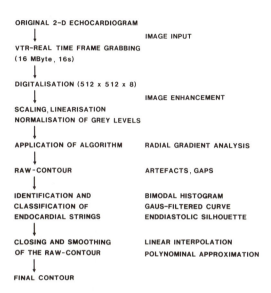

Fig. 4. Flow diagram of automatic contour finding.

ated favorably with the 'true' endocardial contours. The correlation coefficients ranged from r=0.97 to 0.98 and the standard error of the estimate (SEE) was between 0.43 and 0.51 cm². These results compare with the data that Collins and coworkers published in 1984. This group used mainly discriminating techniques and edge enhancement operators for their contour generation. They demonstrated correlations from r=0.90 to 0.92 between their techniques and true endocardial contours [14].

With these animal experiments we were able to demonstrate that in simple geometric figures, such as circles and ellipsoids in short axis slices, automatic and semi-automatic contours could be generated successfully with good correlative and reproducible results compared to 'true' endocardial borders.

In order to prove that automatic contour finding algorithms can also be used in selected and non-selected patients in the clinical setting we applied our contour finding program to a routine patients population [16]. In order to apply the program to apical projections, however, some modifications of the algorithm were necessary.

A flow diagram for automatic contour generation is depicted in Figure 4.

In order to create the image on the data monitor, information is transferred from the magnetic disc to the image memory. Interactive image enhancement techniques such as scaling, linearisation and normalisation of grey levels are performed as described above. On these enhanced images, the automatic contour finding algorithm is applied and creates the 'raw' contour, still containing endo-cardial gaps and artefacts. In the next step the computer identifies and classifies the endocardial string using either a statistical iterative selection procedure, such as a bimodal histogram or more complex procedures such as filtering techniques in time and space domain. After detecting artefacts, endocardial gaps are closed and the raw contour is smoothed by linear interpolation using polynomial approx-imation methods. Following these steps, the computer generates the final contour which is then stored in the computer memory.

The basic concept of the contour finding algorithm is explained in more detail:

Starting from a center point defined by the user, the angular space (0–360 degrees) is divided up into a certain number of rays in a polar coordinate system. Along each of these rays, a set of windows moves radially outwards in steps of one pixel. The width and the heighth of these rectangles are variable. The two windows are positioned vertically on the respective ray and are separated from each other by a gap (N-gap) of the width of the rectangle. For each position of the window, the mean grey value in the inner and outer rectangle is calculated; if the difference (= gradient) between the mean grey value in the outer and in the inner rectangle exceeds a certain threshold value, a contour point is considered to be detected and the corresponding radius (= distance between the position of the window on the ray and the polar origin) is stored (Figure 5).

Classification and identification of endocardial strings is based on the bimodal histogram. The distance of 2 neighbour points is defined as:

$$D = D_{n+1} - D_n \; ;$$

the bimodal histogram plots the relative frequencies of these distances and separates valid from invalid contour points on the basis of the first zero-crossing (Figure 6).

A schematic drawing of the different steps of automatic contour generation with artefact detection and smoothing is shown in Figure 7 a/b.

In a selected patient population of 56 patients we applied this algorithm in apical projections (Figure 8 a/b). The original echocardiograms were graded according to the definition of the left ventricular endocardium, grade I being the best and grade IV being the worst image. In grade I and II echocardiograms left ventricular endocardial contours could be generated automatically in all patients (n = 31), as opposed to group III and IV in which only 15 out of 25 echocardio-grams could be processed automatically.

Endsystolic and enddiastolic volumes, calculated by automatically and man-ually derived contours correlated with r = 0.93 and 0.90 with an SEE of 8.3 and 11.3 ml; the ejection fraction calculated by these two contours showed a correla-tion coefficient of r = 0.93 with an SEE of 5.1%.

In general good correlations between manually and automatically generated contours were found proving the utility of the algorithm in this clinical setting

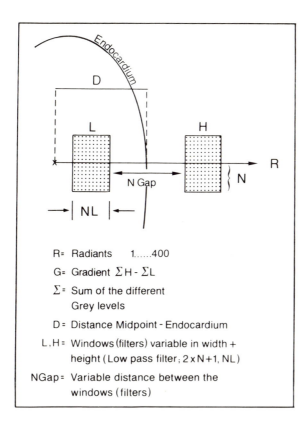

R= Radiants   1.....400

G= Gradient $\Sigma H - \Sigma L$

Σ= Sum of the different
Grey levels

D= Distance Midpoint - Endocardium

L,H= Windows (filters) variable in width +
height (Low pass filter; $2 \times N+1$, NL)

NGap= Variable distance between the
windows (filters)

Fig. 5. Schematic drawing of the computer algorithm for automatic contour detection. Between the two (L and H) rectangles a gradient is calculated which is defined as the difference of the mean grey values of the inner (L) and outer (H) rectangle along up to 400 rays.

(manual versus automatic input of endocardium $r = 0.91$, 0.94; SEE 3.34, 2.77 cm^2). However if the total population is broken up into patients with good and bad quality echocardiograms the interobserver variability and the correlations demonstrate marked differences between the two methods: in the patient group with poor quality echocardiograms the manual input of borders by 2 independent observers revealed a limited correlation ($r = 0.76$) and a large scatter (SEE 5.07 cm^2) as compared to the group with good quality echocardiograms in which the correlations and the scatter are significantly better ($r = 0.97$, SEE 01.95 cm^2).

Automatic generation of endocardial contours in both patients groups revealed overall better correlations, particularly in the group with poor quality echocardiograms (Table 1).

As mentioned before, the detection and elimination of artefacts and the separation between valid and invalid contour points are the most critical steps in automatic contour finding. A bimodal histogram as basis for this procedure can

106

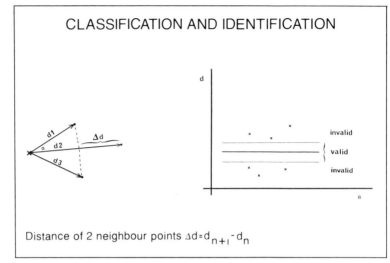

CLASSIFICATION AND IDENTIFICATION

Distance of 2 neighbour points $\Delta d = d_{n+1} - d_n$

A

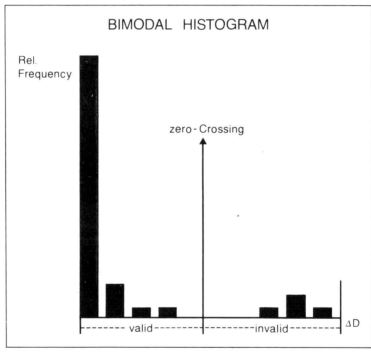

BIMODAL HISTOGRAM

Rel. Frequency

zero-Crossing

-------- valid -------- -------- invalid -------- ΔD

B

Fig. 6 a/b. a) Classification and identification of endocardial strings. The endocardial points P1–P3 have the distance D1–D3 from the center point M to the endocardium. The distance D between two neighbour points are therefore defined as D = D n+1 − Dn. If one plots the distances D against an angle in a polar coordinate system a circle represents a straight line. Within a normal 'band-width' endocardial points will be considered valid and outsine this band as invalid.

b) In a bimodal histogram the relative frequencies of the distances D are plotted as classes; on the basis of the first O-crossing valid and invalid contour points are separated.

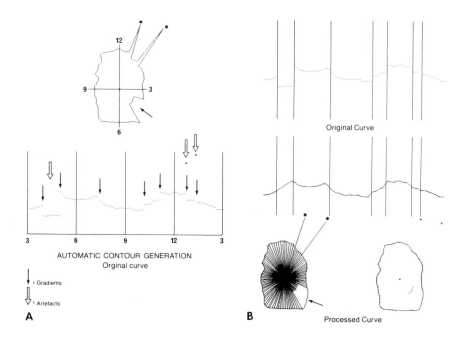

Fig. 7 a/b. a) Schematic drawing of automatic contour generation and artefact detection in a 4-chamber view (upper part). The original contour contains artefacts and endocardial gaps (*). In a polar coordinate system the circumference is divided into 4 quadrants; the x-axis displays the quadrants and the y-axis the distances of the endocardial points from the area mid-point. The arrows mark the gradients and artefacts detected by the computer.

b) The detected gradients and artefacts are marked by vertical lines; in the middle part the 'raw' contour is smoothed and the gaps are closed. In the lower part the final contour is displayed, artefacts are eliminated and endocardial gaps completed.

Table 1. Correlation of LV enddiastolic areas (m²), calculated by manual (man) and automatic (auto) input of endocardial contours by two observers (1, 2). Calculations are made for all echocardiograms (I–IV) as well as for good (I, II) and bad quality echocardiograms.

Qualität	I–IV		I, II		III, IV	
manually n	56		31		25	
automatically(auto) n	44		31		13	
Korrelationen	r	SEE	r	SEE	r	SEE
man 1–man 2	0,87	4,01	0,97	1,95	0,76	5,07
auto 1–auto 2	0,99	0,37	0,99	0,23	0,99	0,57
man 1–auto 1	0,91	3,34	0,94	2,82	0,86	3,65
man 2–auto 2	0,94	2,77	0,96	2,45	0.88	3,38

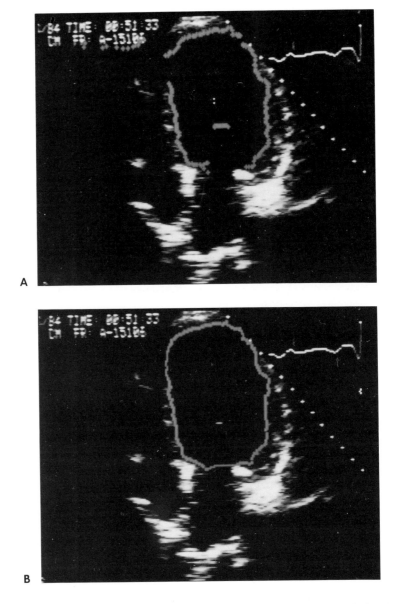

Fig. 8 a/b. The endocardial 'raw'- (a) and final contours in a 4-chamber view are displayed. The 'raw' contour still contains artefacts and gaps, which have been eliminated and closed in the final contour (b).

only be applied to good quality echocardiograms as shown above. It is therefore necessary to develop other modalities of artefact detection; in the following two other methods for artefact detection are proposed and clinically applied:
− the comparison of the raw contour with the Gaussian filtered contour and
− the comparison of each individual contour point or contour string during the cardiac cycle with enddiastolic contour points.
In the latter method all points (pixels) outside the enddiastolic silhouette are a priori considered invalid and are automatically eliminated. This form of artefact detection, however, requires an interactive input of the enddiastolic silhouette.

The former method, particularly useful in poor quality echocardiograms, compares the raw contour with the Gaussian filtered contour; as Gaus filtering suppresses effectively high frequency components of a curve, artefact detection of the 'raw' contour data is accomplished by comparing the 'raw' contour curve with its corresponding Gaussian filtered curve. The root mean square deviation between the raw contour and the Gaussian filtered contour is calculated and every point of the raw contour that deviates more than this root mean square value from the Gaus curve is considered an artefact. Elimination is then completed by linear interpolation.

This method has the advantage that it can be applied both in space- and time domaine as both the spatial distribution of coordinates in one contour curve as well as the motion of one contour point in time have to be reasonably smooth.

Figure 9 depicts a very irregular raw contour in a polar and carthesic coordinate system; multiple artefacts and endocardial gaps are displayed. By overlaying a Gaussian filtered curve (Figure 10) it is obvious that the computer detects the artefacts effectively, suppresses them and closes the endocardial gaps.

This procedure can also be applied in a given contour point at a given angle 'phi' and followed throughout the cardiac cycle so that filtering and artefact detection can be accomplished both in time- and space domaine. In the final contour the artefacts are suppressed and the endocardial gaps are filled.

We examined this procedure in 128 randomly selected patients with various heart diseases. 40 patients had cardiomyopathies, 56 patients had coronary heart disease and 32 patients had valvular heart disease. We graded the 2-dimensional echocardiograms according to the quality of endocardial definition by two observers. Grade I constitued a group in which the endocardial borders were totally defined and grade II were patients in whom the endocardial borders were only partially defined but easy to complete. Grade III and IV were echocardiograms of minor quality in which the endocardial definition was insufficient and difficult to complete and were filled with intra- and extracavitary artefacts as well as with large endocardial drop-outs.

After selecting the appropriate cardiac cycles for evaluation from a video tape recorder, endsystolic and enddiastolic frames were depicted by two observers and the endocardial outlines were drawn manually via an X-Y tablet and determined

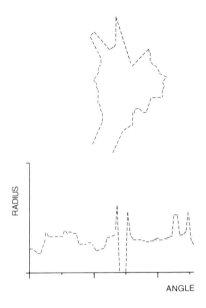

Fig. 9. Schematic drawing of a endocardial raw contour of a poor quality echocardiogramm in a carthesic and polar coordinate system (dashed line). Note the artefacts and gaps.

automatically using the contour finding algorithm. Artefact elimination was performed by comparing the original curve with the Gaus-filtered curve and by the bimodal histogram. Enddiastolic and endsystolic volumes as well as wall motion parameters were calculated using five areas in a fixed extracardiac reference system for evaluation. In addition we compared the results of the two observers thus establishing the interobserver variability (in %).

In all echocardiograms with good endocardial definition (grade I and II; n = 31, 55%), in 29 patients of group III and in 7 patients of group IV we were able to generate the endocardial contour automatically using various pre-processing steps particularly in poor quality echocardiograms. In 9 patients of group III and in 10 patients of group IV automatic contour finding was not successful because endocardial gaps were larger than 30% of the total endocardial circumference. LV volumes and ejection fraction calculated on the basis of manually and automatically generated contours correlated favorably (r = 0.90–0.93 and SEE between 8.3 and 11.3 ml and 5.4%) thus demonstrating good agreement between the two methods. Despite these correlations, however, manual input of borders caused marked differences in interobserver variability (V) depending upon the echocardiographic image quality: in patients with complete endocardial definition (grade I and II) the reproducibility was superior (V = 3.0–4.0, SD = 2.81–3.12) to echocardiograms with poor and incomplete endocardial definition (V = 9.8–15.2, SD of 4.24–6.10); these results are in contrast to automatic contour finding regardless of the original echocardiographic quality: V = 0.40 and 0.99, SD = 1.10 and 0.28. These results demonstrate that automatic contour definition,

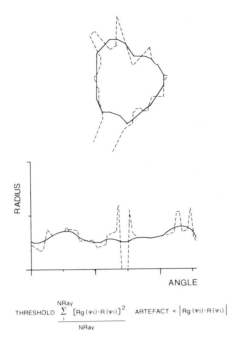

$$\text{THRESHOLD} \quad \frac{\overset{NRay}{\underset{i}{\Sigma}} [Rg(\psi_i)-R(\psi_i)]^2}{NRay} \qquad \text{ARTEFACT} < \left| Rg(\psi_i)-R(\psi_i) \right|$$

Fig. 10. The same raw contour as in figure 9 with overlay of the corresponding Gaus filtered contour (continuous line). The artefacts are detected and the gaps are closed by linear interpolation.

Table 2. Reproducibility of left ventricular function parameters, calculated on the basis of manually (man) and automatically (auto) generated contours.

	Qualität	I–IV		I, II		III, IV	
		V	SD	V	SD	V	SD
EDF	man 1–man 2	8,5	6,52	4,0	3,0	14,1	5,31
(cm²)	auto 1–auto 2	0,63	0,62	0,49	0,33	0,95	0,96
ESF	man 1–man 2	6,3	4,32	3,5	2,81	10,2	4,24
(cm²)	auto 1–auto 2	0,60	0,58	0,34	0,30	0,79	0,68
EDV	man 1–man 2	8,1	6,52	3,9	2,91	15,2	6,10
(ml)	auto 1–auto 2	0,66	0,59	0,52	0,41	0,99	1,10
ESV	man 1–man 2	5,9	4,76	3,0	2,99	9,8	5,16
(ml)	auto 1–auto 2	0,57	0,43	0,45	0,28	0,86	0,80
EF	man 1–man 2	4,8	3,98	3,8	3,12	12,6	5,62
(%)	auto 1–auto 2	0,68	0,54	0,40	0,32	0,89	0,76

EDF, ESF = enddiastolic and endsystolic areas. EDV, ESV = enddiastolic and endsystolic volumes. EF = ejection fraction. V and SD denote the mean and the standard deviation of the reproducibility (agreement of results between two observers).

particularly in echocardiograms with minor quality, improves the reproducibility and therefore the diagnostic safety of this procedure.

The results of the reproducibilities are shown in Table 2.

Despite encouraging results of automatic contour finding with various complex computer algorithms, there are some limitations that have to considered and possibly prevent these methods from wide-spread clinical application:

1. Computer algorithms for automatic edge detection are usually part of complex and complicated software developments;
2. These algorithms can usually not be used in all echocardiographic projections such as in short axis and in apical views without modifications and they are dependent of the echocardiographic image quality.
3. The application of the algorithms needs some understanding for computer technology and
4. its successful use needs research work by skilled personel.
5. Complex computer algorithms usually only work on high technology computers and therefore need a certain amount of financial investment.

We therefore looked for less complicated and less expensive alternatives for automatic edge detection methods. *Digital subtraction echocardiography* (DSE) of contrast echocardiograms fulfills most of the requirements for safe and reproducible endocardial detection in echocardiograms. The hardware and software requirements are, compared to the use of computer algorithms, minimal and almost no skill of the observer is needed for evaluation [22, 23].

A flow scheme of digital subtraction echocardiography is shown in Figure 11.

A prerequisite for the successful application of digital subtraction echocardiography is the homogeneous and complete opacification of the cardiac chambers in order to achieve clear delineation of the endocardial surface. Conventional contrast agents such as saline, glucose, indocyanine green, CO_2 or H_2O_2 allow qualitative analysis of intracardiac flow characteristics such as in shunts or regurgitation; a quantitative analysis of left ventricular function parameters, however, are not possible because these contrast agents fail to opacify the cardiac chamber completely.

New echo-contrast agents such as oxypolygelatine or SH U 454 can be applied safely and lead to a homogeneous contrast of the cardiac chamber (Figure 12b) [24, 25]; in analogy to digital subtraction angiography the most important step in DSE is the subtraction of digitized grey level information of an original echocardiogram from a phase-identical contrast image (masc-mode subtraction) (Figure 12c).

By this technique the endocardium, as the most important intracardiac structure for the calculation of left and right ventricular function parameters, is displayed as the borderline of the contrast depot (Figure 12e) [26].

In order to calculate the reproducibility of endocardial definition by different evaluation methods such as digital subtraction echocardiography, automatic

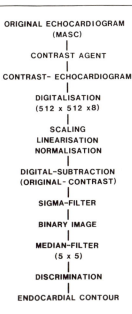

Fig. 11. Flow scheme of digital subtraction echocardiography.

computer algorithm and conventional manual input of endocardial borders and in order to test some conventional and newer echo-contrast agents for their use in digital subtraction echocardiography we performed animal studies with 10 Beagle dogs [22]. The dogs were anesthetized and their heart was displayed in a modified 4-chamber view from a parasternal transducer position. With a fixed transducer postion echocontrast agents were injected as a bolus through an indwelling saphenous vein catheter. 2 ml of each contrast medium (0.9% saline, indocyanine green (ICG), H_2O_2, CO_2, Haemaccel, SH U 454) was injected maximally 3 times and the examination was stored on video tape for later evaluation.

Left ventricular endocardium in the original- and contrast-echocardiograms was defined manually by tracing the endocardial outline with a cursor on an X-Y tablet by 2 independent observers. Automatic contour detection in original echocardiograms was performed by the previously described complex computer algorithm; in contrast echocardiograms endocardial boders were defined by digital subtraction techniques and grey level discrimination.

The complete echocardiographic examination was stored on video tape and evaluated off-line by a commercially available evaluation computer (MIP-Kardio 2000, Firma KONTRON Bildanalyse, Eching bei München). Appropriate echo-cardiographic frames were selected and digitized in a $512 \times 512 \times 8$ bit grey level matrix (Figure 12 a/b). Following image pre-processing by scaling, linearisation

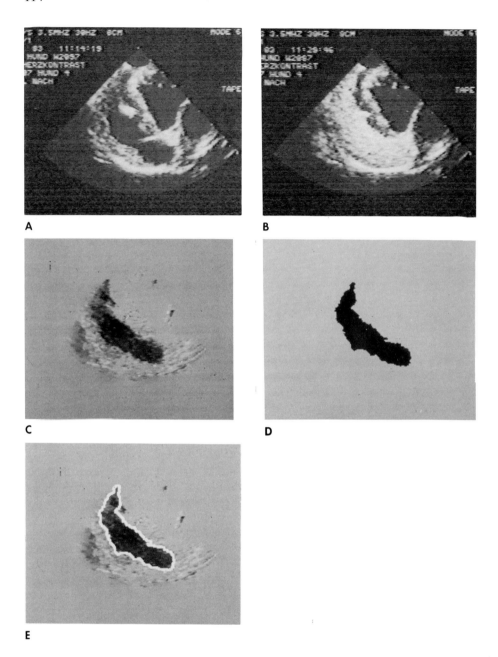

Fig. 12 a–e. Original (a) and contrast echocardiogram (b) in a modified 4-chamber view of an anesthetized dog with SH U 454. Digital subtraction of the original echocardiogram from its corresponding, phase identical contrast image results in a digital subtraction echocardiogram (DSE) (c), in which the contrast depot within the right ventricular chamber is distinctly diplayed in dark colors. The binary image (d) serves as basis for the definition of endocardium, which is shown around the contrast depot in the DSE.

and normalisation of grey levels a SIGMA-filter was used in order to eliminate the background noise. Digital subtraction of the original echocardiogram from its corresponding, phase identical contrast image was then performed (Figure 12c).

In a digital subtraction echocardiogram the cardiac structures such as myocardium and valves are displayed in weak, light grey colors, whereas the contrast depot within the cardiac chamber is displayed in dark-shaded colors with clearly defined endocardial edges.

The next step consisted of grey level discrimination and conversion into a black and white binary image (Figure 12d); this image served as the basis for the definition of endocardium. The program for endocardial definition is based on the detection of black and white grey level differences between the ventricular cavity and myocardial tissue. The computer stores these border points as X-Y coordinates and the complete string then represents the continuous endocardial border (Figure 12e).

The results of the different evaluation methods were compared with each other and the areas enclosed by these borders served as basis for the calculation of reproducibility (in %) and correlations.

Our studies revealed that digital subtraction echocardiograms could not be generated with saline, CO_2 and 1% H_2O_2 because these contrast media were unable to completely opacify the cardiac chambers. Indocyanine green and haemaccel demonstrated sufficient results as compared to the manual input of endocardial borders. The correlation coefficients and the standard error of the estimate ranged between $r = 0.85$ and 0.89 and 3.98 and $1.00 \, cm^2$. The best correlations were found with SH U 454 a new echo-contrast agent containing saccharose-stabilised micro-bubbles with a size of below 6.5 (median 3.0). In concentrations between 100 and 300 mg/ml correlation coefficients were in the range of $r = 0.95$ and 0.98 with an SEE of 0.21 and $0.56 \, cm^2$ between manually and automatically (by DSE) derived contours.

Comparing the different results of the reproducibility studies we found with manual input of endocardial borders in original echocardiograms values between 12.3% and 16.9%. Manual input of endocardium in contrast-echocardiograms revealed better results because of better delineation of these borders by contrast agents; interobserver variabilities ranged between 2.0% (SH U 454 300 mg/ml) and 15.7% (CO_2). Automatic definition of endocardium by digital subtraction echocardiography revealed the best results with reproducibilities between 0.9% (SH U 454, 300 mg/ml) and 7.6% (0.5% ICG).

Our animal experiments showed, that digital subtraction echocardiography is a simple and safe procedure to define endocardial contours if echo-contrast media lead to an uniform and homogeneous opacification of the cardiac chambers. Only SH U 454 and haemaccel seem to be appropriate for this purpose and result in good correlations between manually and automatically derived endocardial contours with good reproducibility of data. The combined use of digital subtraction echocardiography and appropriate contrast media therefore seem to enhance the safety and accuracy of endocardial definition and consequently of quantitative evaluation of ventricular function parameters.

In order to define the *clinical utility* of digital subtraction echocardiography we determined left ventricular function parameters, such as volumes and ejection fraction, in a routine patient population of 57 consecutive patients undergoing diagnostic left heart catheterisation [23]. 33 patients had coronary heart disease, 11 patients had valvular heart disease, 12 patients had congestive cardiomyopathies and 1 patient had coarctation of the aorta. We injected 2–4 ml of 5.5% oxypolygelatine (Gelifundol S) as bolus into the left ventricle through an indwelling pig-tail angiographic catheter.

Echocardiographic determinations of left ventricular ejection fraction, enddiastolic and endsystolic volumes, were achieved by manual definition of endocardial borders in original and contrast echocardiograms (Figure 13 a/b) and by digital subtraction echocardiography (Figure 14 a/b). These results were then compared with the invasive cardiac catheterisation data.

Digital subtraction echocardiography was performed the same way as described previously in animal experiments except for triggering of echocardiographic frames in endsystole and enddiastole using the R-wave of the electrocardiogram as trigger signal.

In 57 consecutive patients we determined left ventricular ejection fraction as well as volumes of the left ventricle echocardiographically and cineangiographically. The results of the angiographically calculated ejection fraction and volumes of all 57 patients served as 'gold standard'.

We were able to perform a quantitative analysis of left ventricular function in the original 2-D echocardiogram by manual input of endocardial borders in 49 patients (87%). In 8 patients (12.3%) the endocardial definition was insufficient for outlining these borders. In contrast to original echocardiograms we were able to quantify left ventricular function in all patients with contrast echocardiograms because of clear endocardial delineation by the contrast agents.

In 44 patients (77.2%) digital subtraction techniques could be applied due to the uniform and homogeneous opacification of the left cardiac chamber with complete outline of the endo-myocardial border. In 13 patients we were not able to perform digital subtraction echocardiography because the left ventricle was insufficiently contrasted or because the indwelling pig-tail catheter caused strong reflections that could not be decreased by various filtering techniques.

Echocardiographically calculated endsystolic volumes demonstrated a better correlation with invasive volumes (r = 0.88, and r = 0.85) than enddiastolic volumes (r = 0.76 and r = 0.78). The SEE was larger in enddiastolic volumes (41.4 and 39.6 ml) than in endsystolic volumes wit an SEE of 22.5 and 24.6 ml as a consequence of better endocardial reflection properties in endsystole.

Ventricular ejection fraction calculated on the basis of automatic contour definition by digital subtraction techniques demonstrated better correlations with angiographic data (r = 0.89, SEE 5.8% in 44 patients) (Figure 15), than manual

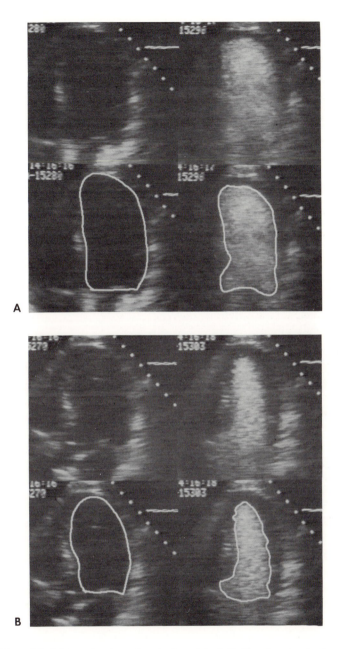

Fig. 13 a/b. Manual definition of endocardium in the original- (left) and contrast-echocardiogramm (right) of a 4-chamber view in enddiastole (a) and in endsystole (b). The left ventricular cavity is completely opacified by the contrast agent (5.5% oxypolygelatine) and therefore the endocardial border can easily be marked. In the original echocardiogram the endocardial borders are markedly overestimated compared to the contrast-echocardiogram, because the 'true' endocardium is not visualized. In the contrast images the 'halo-effect' (echo-free endo-myocardium) is distinctly displayed.

118

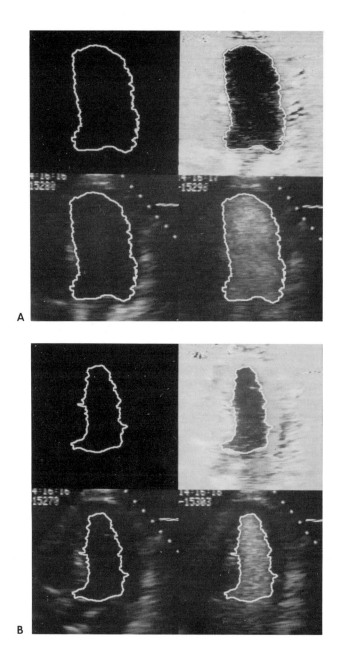

Fig. 14 a/b. Enddiastolic (a) and endsystolic silhouettes (b) automatically generated by digital subtraction echocardiography (upper right). These silhouettes are projected into the original- (lower left) and contrast echocardiogramm (lower right). It is obvious that the echo-free border zone of the myocardium, not visualized in the original echocardiogram is marked-off against the left ventricular cavity.

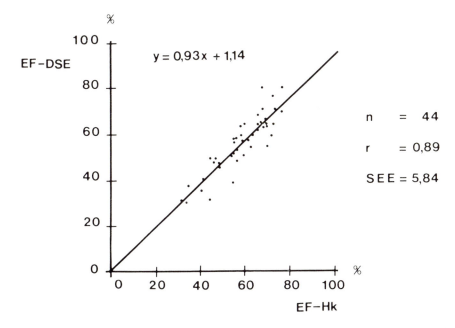

Fig. 15. Correlation of the ejection fraction calculated by digital subtraction echocardiography (EF-DSE) and by angiography (EF-HK).

endocardial input of original echocardiograms with r = 0.71, SEE 8.1% in 47 patients (Figure 16). Good correlations were also found between the ejection fraction calculated on the basis of manual input of endocardial borders of contrast echocardiograms and invasively determined ejection fraction with r = 0.92, SEE 4.3%.

On the basis of these calculations we conclude, that the ejection fraction by digital subtraction echocardiography and contrast echocardiograms approaches the results of the invasive data as opposed to the ejection fraction calculated by original echocardiography.

As has been known from previous studies [3, 6] echocardiographic volumes and ejection fraction markedly underestimate cardiac catheterisation data due to inherent systematic errors.

Additionally in original echocardiograms the endocardial borders are sometimes unprecise and incomplete, so that calculations of volumes, ejection fraction and wall motion, even by experienced observers are often unreliable. In contrast-echocardiograms, however, left ventricular cavities are completely opacified and endocardial borders are precisely delineated so that calculations are reproducible and reliable.

Digital subtraction echocardiography uses these advantages of echo-contrast ventriculography by means of automatic definition on the basis of grey level discrimination. The calculation of LV function parameters, in particular the

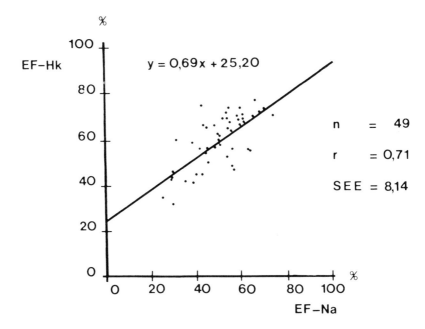

Fig. 16. Correlation of the ejection fraction calculated by the original echocardiogram (EF-NA) and by angiography (EF-HK).

ejection fraction, are reproducible and independent of echocardiographic image qualities and of the subjective experience of the observer.

We conclude from our studies, that digital subtraction echocardiography is a simple and safe method to define 'true' endocardial borders of the right and the left ventricle. Analysis of left ventricular function parameters such as volumes and ejection fraction, revealed good correlations with invasive, angiographic data. Therefore the diagnostic safety and the clinical value of 2-D contrast-echocardiography is greatly increased. Some limitations in the use of digital subtraction techniques have to be considered, however:

– conventional echo-contrast agents are inadequate for the complete opacification of the ventricular cavity so that quantitative evaluation of LV function is not possible and

– digital subtraction can only be performed with images in digitized format so that this technique is dependent on computers with an adequate image memory.

References

1. Moynihan PF, Parisi AF, Feldmann CL: Quantitative detection of regional left ventricular contraction abnormalities by two-dimensional echocardiography. Circulation 1981; 63: 752.
2. Parisi AF, Moynihan PF, Folland ED, Feldman CL: Quantitative detection of regional ventricular contraction abnormalities by two-dimensional echocardiography. Circulation 1981; 63: 761.
3. Rein AJJT, Sapoznikov D, Lewis N, Halon DA, Gotsman MS, Lewis BS: Regional left ventricular ejection fraction from realtime two-dimensional echocardiography. Int J Cardiol 1982; 2:61.
4. Erbel R, Schweizer P, Lambertz H, Henn G, Meyer J, Krebs W, Effert S: Echoventriculography. A simultaneous analysis of two-dimensional echocardiography and cineventriculography. Circulation 1983; 67: 205.
5. Erbel R, Schweizer P, Pyel N, Harde U, Meyer J, Effert S: Quantitative Analyse regionaler Kontraktionsstörungen des linken Ventrikels im zweidimensionalen Echokardiogramm. Z Kardiol 1980; 69: 562.
6. Folland ED, Parisi AF, Moynihan BS, Jones DR: Assessment of left ventricular volumes and ejection fraction by real time two dimensional echocardiography. Circulation 1979; 60: 670.
7. Grube E, Hanisch H, Neumann G, Simon H: Quantitative evaluation of LV wall motion by two-dimensional echocardiography. J Am Coll Cardiol 1983; 1(2): 581.
8. Grube E, Backs B, Hanisch H, Zywietz M, Neumann G: Quantitative rechnergestützte Bestimmung linksventrikulärer Kontraktionsanomalien im zweidimensionalen Echokardiogramm. II. Anwendung bei Patienten mit koronarer Herzkrankheit. Z Kardiol 1984; 73: 71.
9. Kisslo JA, Robertson W, Gilbert BW, v.Ramm O, Behar VS: A comparison of real-time two dimensional echocardiography and cineangiography in detecting left ventricular asynergy. Circulation 1977; 5: 134.
10. Grube E, Richter R, Otten H, Janson R, Lackner K, Simon H, Jörgens H: Darstellung linksventrikulärer Kontraktionsanomalien mit Hilfe der zweidimensionalen Sektor Echokardiographie. Dtsch Med Wschr 1979; 104: 703.
11. Erbel R: personal communication 1985.
12. Grube E, Hanisch H, Zywietz M, Neumann G, Herzog H: Rechnergestützte Bestimmung linksventrikulärer Kontraktionsanomalien mittels zweidimensionaler Echokardiographie. I. Analyse verschiedener Untersuchungsmethoden und Normalwertbestimmung. Z Kardiol 1984; 73: 41.
13. Budal AI, Delp EJ, Meyer CR, Jenkins JM, Smith DN, Bookstein FL, Pitt B: Automatic computer processing of digital 2-dimensional echocardiograms. Am J Cardiol 1983; 52: 384.
14. Collins SM, Skorton DJ et al: Computer assisted edge detection in two-dimensional echocardiography: comparison with anatomic data. Am J Cardiol 1984; 53: 1380.
15. Garcia E, Gueret P, Bennett M, Corday E, Zwehl W, Meerbaum S, Corday S, Swan HJC: Real-time computerisation of two-dimensional echocardiography. Am Heart J 1981; 101: 763.
16. Grube E, Backs A, Backs B, Lüderitz B: Automatische Konturerkennung im zweidimensionalen Echokardiogramm. Untersuchungen an einem allgemeinen Patientenkollektiv. Z Kardiol 1985; 74: 445.
17. Grube E, Nitsch J, Backs B: Automatic border extraction from 2-D echocardiograms. Circulation 1983; Suppl 23: 43.
18. Grube E, Mathers F, Backs B, Lüderitz B: Automatische und halbautomatische Konturfindung des linken Ventrikels im zweidimensionalen Echokardiogramm. In-vitro-Untersuchungen an formalinfixierten Schweineherzen. Z Kardiol 1985; 74: 15.
19. Skorton DJ, McNary CA, Child JS, Newton FC, Shah PM: Digital image processing of two dimensional echocardiograms: identification of endocardium. Am J Cardiol 1981; 48: 479.
20. Zwehl W, Levy R et al: Validation of a computerized edge detection algorithm for quantitative two-dimensional echocardiography. Circulation 1984; 68: 1127.
21. Melton HE, Collins SM, Skorton DJ: Automatic real-time endocardial edge detection during two-dimensional echocardiographic examination. Circulation 1982; Suppl II: 337.

22. Grube E, Fritzsch T: Verbesserte Reproduzierbarkeit der Kontrasttechnokardiographie durch SH U 454. Experimentelle Untersuchungen mittels digitaler Subtraktionsechokardiographie. Z Kardiol 1986; (in press).
23. Grube E, Lampen M, Becher H: Echokontrast-Ventrikulographie. Bestimmung linksventrikulärer Funktionsparameter unter besonderer Berücksichtigung der digitalen Subtraktionsechokardiographie. Z Kardiol 1986; (in press).
24. Smith MD, Kwan OL, Reiser HJ, DeMaria AN: Superior intensity and reproducibility of SH U 454, a new right heart contrast agent. J Am Coll Cardiol 1984; 3: 992.
25. Fritsch T, Lange L, Schartel M, Hilman J, Rasor J, Reiser J: The characteristics of the new safe non-lung crossing echocontrast agent SH U 454 for reproducible and homogeneous opacification of blood and myocardium. Eur Heart J 1984; 5: 197.
26. Wann LS, Stickels KR, Bannrah VS, Gross CM: Digital processing of contrast echocardiograms: a new technique for measuring right ventricular ejection fraction. Am J Cardiol 1984; 53: 1164.

9. Digitised M-Modes – the Clinical Yield

R.J.C. HALL
Royal Victoria Infirmary, Newcastle upon Tyne, UK

Digitisation of the M-mode echocardiogram is the use of a simple combination of a digitising tablet and computer to make measurements from the M-mode tracing. It is a way of facilitating measurement of simple variables such as chamber dimensions and wall thickness and of obtaining more complex measurements such as rates of change of those variables (Figure 1). When M-mode was the only way in which echocardiograms could be presented, digitisation to obtain these more complex variables often added to the useful clinical information obtained [1] e.g. in the assessment of valve disease (see below). Nowadays with the advent of high quality cross-sectional images and Doppler techniques many of these clinically useful applications have been superceded. Digitisation of M-mode tracings however produced considerable advances in the understanding of left ventricular function in a way that is still impossible from these newer techniques [1]. M-mode remains the only really accurate way of assessing cavity dimensions and timing cardiac events and the combination of these two attributes lead to the development of the concept of left ventricular inco-ordination which is the hallmark of disturbances of left ventricular function associated with ischaemic heart disease [1, 2, 3]. Similarly its ability to allow detailed study of diastolic events such as rates of change of dimension and wall thickness both during isovolumic relaxation and the later phases of diastole has focussed attention on the importance of this phase of the cardiac cycle [4].

Much of the clinical information derived from both M-mode and cross-sectional echocardiography is at best semi-quantitative and often qualitative. Sophisticated measurements are not required to tell normal from very poor left function, very severe from very mild mitral stenosis, or the presence or absence of vegetations or thrombus within the heart. Measurement, of which digitisation can be regarded as a sophisticated variety, is necessary when trying to assess problems of moderate or doubtful severity or when following sequential changes, e.g. the progressive change of LV dimension in aortic regurgitation.

If a technique is to be used in this way its reproducibility must be known. Research studies often compare data derived from groups of patients and show significant differences in a variable between the groups, e.g. the peak rate of LV

J. Roelandt (editor), *Digital Techniques in Echocardiography*. ISBN 0-89838-861-9.
© 1987, Martinus Nijhoff Publishers, Dordrecht. Printed in the Netherlands.

124

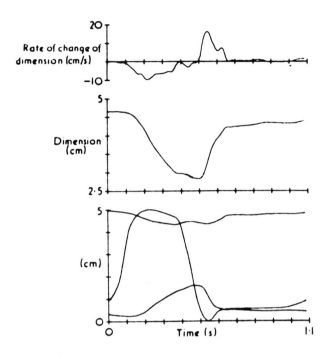

Fig. 1. Digitised echocardiogram from a normal subject (and a simultaneous apexcardiogram). The lower panel is the tracing of the original echocardiogram. The middle panel shows the left ventricular dimension and the upper panel shows the first derivative of the middle panel, i.e. the rate of change of dimension. Note the initial rapid dimension change in diastole.

diastolic dimension change in mild and severe mitral stenosis [5] (Figure 2), or correlate such a variable with another well established technique e.g. the valve area derived at catheterisation [6]. The problem with both methods is that it is difficult or impossible to apply this type of data to individual patients. In the individual patient it is the reproducibility and 95% confidence limits of a single measurement that are relevant but these are not defined by group studies where the individual variability of measurements is submerged by the process of obtaining group means. Initial studies of digitisation suggested that variations in measurement are insignificant but subsequent studies have shown that this is not the case [7]. These studies emphasise that, not surprisingly, measurements from very high quality tracings are considerably more accurate than those from poor tracings and therefore all echocardiographic departments should strive for high quality images and discard those of poor quality. Unfortunately this is not always the case and sophisticated measurements made from poor tracings are worse than useless since they lead to a disillusionment with the technique which is unjustified. Although there have been studies of the reproducibility of measurements in normals [7] the same techniques have not been applied in the same detail to abnormals. This may be important since the degree of reproducibility may be

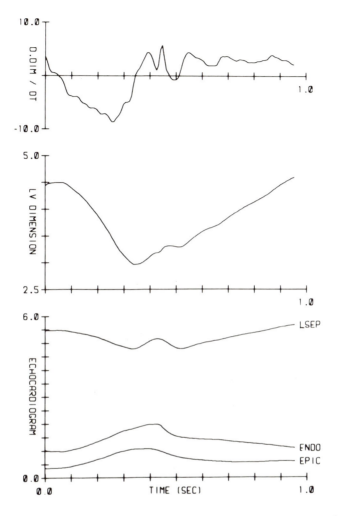

Fig. 2. Digitised echocardiogram in mitral stenosis. The format is as in Figure 1. Note the slow left ventricular dimension change in diastole and the lack of a rapid filling period. LSEP = left side of septum, ENDO = endocardium, EPI = epicardium.

greater and the 95% confidence limits narrower in certain circumstances. A good example is the assessment of reduced peak rate of LV diastolic dimension change in mitral stenosis. The slower rate of LV dimension change in mitral stenosis should theoretically be easier to measure accurately than the faster rate in normals. There are other ways to narrow the confidence limits of a variable. The most useful is to simply repeat the measurement and take the mean. Although this technique is often used to eliminate beat to beat variation there is another reason for doing it since it has been shown that replication error by the digitiser (i.e. the inability to digitise the same tracing in exactly the same way each time) is the main source of error in digitisation [7]. Such an observation, established in the realm of digitisation, is probably true for most other forms of measurement.

Another problem that besets all types of measurement, including digitisation, is the necessity for appropriate controls. Unfortunately control values used in published or clinical work are often inadequate e.g. data obtained from text books, physically fit medical students or hospital staff or from other centres are often used. They rarely take into account the age, sex, body size or race of the patients which are compared to the control group.

Despite these problems with measurement and the advent of new techniques, digitised M-mode echocardiograms still have a small but useful place in clinical practice.

Valve disease

Mitral lesions produce characteristic changes in left ventricular behaviour. These changes are not always specific to these conditions but particularly if absent may sometimes arouse suspicions about the diagnosis and lead to careful reassessment. Mitral stenosis and to some extent prosthetic mitral valves disturb left ventricular filling (Figure 2). In mitral stenosis groups of patients with mild and severe stenosis can be distinguished by the rate at which left ventricular dimension changes during diastole, and the presence or absence of a period of rapid left ventricular filling in early diastole [5]. Because of the problems of wide 95% confidence limits for measurements in individual patients referred to above, these measurements can never give a completely accurate measurement of the severity of stenosis. However if rapid LV filling is seen in a patient in whom severe stenosis is suspected or slow filling is seen in a patient with suspected mild disease, then complete reassessment, if necessary by cardiac catheterisation, is needed. Similarly patients with significant mitral regurgitation usually have hyperdynamic left ventricles and an increased rate of left ventricular dimension change [1] (Figure 3). If the digitised M-mode fails to reveal this then the diagnosis needs serious reconsideration. Figure 4 shows the peak rates of left ventricular filling in several groups of patients with valve disease.

One of the most useful applications of the digitised M-mode is in the diagnosis of mitral prosthetic valve dysfunction [8, 9]. All mitral prostheses even when functioning normally, severely restrict the flow of blood into the left ventricle in diastole. Mechanical prostheses in general do this more than biological prostheses. When mitral prostheses leak the physical signs are often difficult to interpret [10]. Particularly when the leak is paraprosthetic there may be no murmur and the patient may present with unexplained heart failure. In all patients with prosthetic valves in whom a clinical deterioration occurs, prosthetic valve dysfunction must be eliminated as a cause before some other explanation of the deterioration is accepted. Two features on the M-mode echocardiogram may

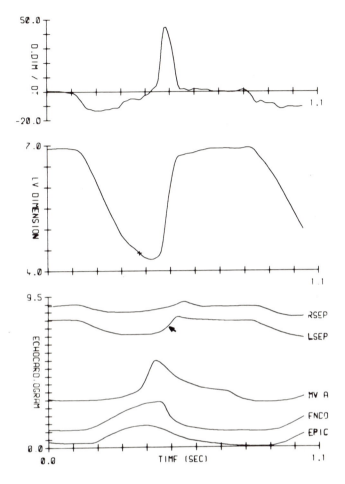

Fig. 3. Digitised echocardiogram in mitral regurgitation. The format is as in Figure 1. Note the very rapid early diastolic dimension change. The arrow shows the characteristic early septal motion seen in mitral regurgitation. LSEP and RSEP = left and right side of septum, ENDO and EPI = endo and epicardium, MVA is the anterior cusp of the mitral valve.

be helpful. Firstly nearly all patients with mitral Starr-Edwards prostheses which are functioning normally and most patients with disc valves have reversed septal motion [10]. A significant paraprosthetic leak often causes septal motion to revert to normal [10]. Secondly the peak rate of LV diastolic dimension change is moderately reduced in patients with prosthetic mitral valves but when a significant leak occurs it returns to the normal or supra-normal values [8, 9]. The M-mode echocardiogram is not particularly helpful when there is prosthetic valve obstruction since although the LV filling rate may fall somewhat in the individual patient, this fall is small and occurs from an already low rate [11]. Clinical signs such as the absence of mechanical valve clicks and radiographic or cross-sectional

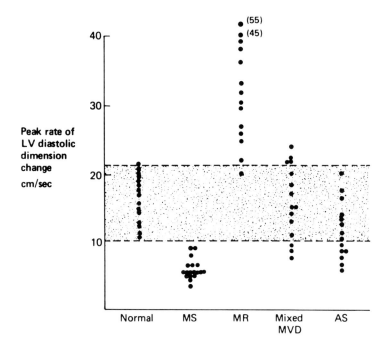

Fig. 4. Peak left ventricular dimension change in normals, mitral stenosis (MS), mitral regurgitation (MR), mixed mitral valve disease (mixed MVD) and aortic stenosis (AS). The cross hatched area represents the normal range.

evidence of reduced ball, disc or cusp motion are much more useful. Poor LV function does not dramatically change rates of LV diastolic dimension change and therefore the digitised M-mode can distinguish these patients from those with significant paraprosthetic leaks but not from those with obstructed valves [9].

The digitised M-mode has a much more limited yield in aortic valve disease. Serial measurements of LV dimension are useful in following the progression of aortic regurgitation although the correct point at which to intervene surgically remains undefined. Such measurements are best made from the M-mode but do not really require recourse to digitisation. More complex disturbances of LV function which can be detected by the digitised M-mode occur in aortic valve disease [14], but are not as easily applied to clinical practice as those obtained in mitral valve disease. If 'isovolumic' relaxation is defined by e.g. the interval between the aortic component of second heart sound recorded on a simultaneous phonocardiogram and mitral valve opening or the downstroke of a simultaneously recorded apexcardiogram there is an increase in LV dimension during this period in patients with aortic regurgitation. This occurs because regurgitation through the aortic valve begins as soon as ejection ends and thus before 'isovolumic relaxation' has had a chance to take place. Although this is a striking physiological finding it has little or no clinical use.

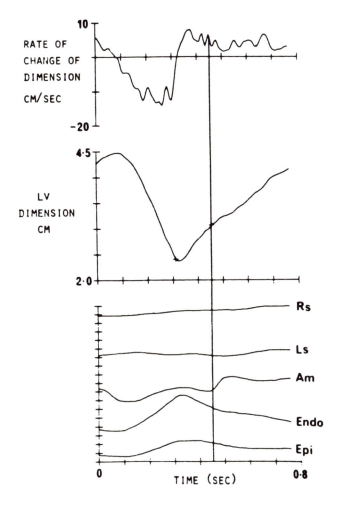

Fig. 5. Digitised echocardiogram in aortic stenosis. The format is as in Figure 1. Note the slow left ventricular peak rate of dimension change and marked left ventricular hypertrophy. Ls and Rs = left and right sides of septum, Am = anterior cusp of the mitral valve. Endo and Epi = endo and epicardium.

The most consistent change in aortic stenosis is a reduced LV filling rate (Figure 5). This is not specific or invariable and is seen in most types of prolonged severe hypertrophy and is probably the result of changes in the properties of the hypertrophied muscle [12]. There is no direct correlation of this abnormality and the severity of stenosis but it is important to recognise its existence since it may cause confusion when trying to assess LV filling in combined aortic and mitral valve disease.

Left ventricular disease

The main problem of using the M-mode echocardiogram, digitised or undigitised, in the assessment of the left ventricle is the very limited view of the base of the left ventricle obtained with this technique. The introduction of cross-sectional echo-cardiography which displays the whole ventricle does not have this drawback in the 70% or so of patients in whom good images can be obtained. It is generally a preferable technique for assessing overall left ventricular function although it may easily miss subtle abnormalities of function that can be detected by disturbed timing of wall motion on the digitised M-mode tracing [3]. The commonest and most easily recognised of these abnormalities consist of delayed mitral valve opening due to prolongation of isovolumic relaxation and abnormal (usually outward) wall motion before the mitral valve opens. This latter sign of left ventricular inco-ordination represents a change in left ventricular shape]1]. Somewhere outside the M-mode beam part of the ventricle moves inward rapidly before the mitral valve opens because the function of the segment is disturbed by ischaemia. Since the ventricle cannot change volume before the mitral valve opens another part of the ventricle (often the basal part seen by the M-mode) has to move outwards. This small change of timing with wall motion occurring before the mitral valve opens will not be obvious from the cross-sectional recording but has important physiological effects [13] on the circulation since this wall motion is not used for ventricular filling. Although this type of analysis of LV function from digitised M-modes is most useful for research it occasionally suggests a clinical diagnosis of myocardial ischaemia which has not been detected in another way.

The best way of diagnosing left ventricular aneurysm non-invasively is with cross-sectional echocardiography. For the unfortunate clinician with only M-mode the digitised M-mode may help make the diagnosis [14]. Relatively preserved basal contraction with obvious evidence of LV inco-ordination due to the aneurysm are the main features (delay in mitral valve opening > 80 msec; normal < 40 msec; fractional shortening $> 25\%$ and end systolic dimension of base of LV > 5.5 cms).

Although the digitised M-mode is often extremely abnormal in cardiomyopathy these changes are usually non-specific and of no clinical use. There is however one situation in which the digitised M-mode is sometimes very helpful. Amyloid cardiomyopathy make up between 5 and 10% of all cardiomyopathies of non-ischaemic origin [15], therefore although rare in general practice, is seen quite frequently by cardiologists. It is often easily diagnosed from the brilliant, scintillating echoes that the amyloid laden myocardium generates but on occasions this is not particularly obvious. In these circumstances the problem is to distinguish the myocardial thickening it produces by infiltration from left ventricular hypertrophy. The digitised M-mode helps in this differentiation [15]. Although the peak rate of left ventricular diastolic dimension change is somewhat reduced in hypertrophy (see above) amyloid infiltration reduces it even further.

The pattern of this reduction is different from that seen in mitral stenosis. In amyloid the early phase of LV filling is not prolonged but the rate of filling is reduced during this phase and there then follows a period of diastasis. In severe mitral stenosis the rate of early LV filling is similarly reduced but filling continues slowly throughout diastole without diastasis occurring [5].

Conclusions

The use of digitised M-mode has had a major impact on understanding LV function particularly in ischaemic heart disease. The technique still has a small clinical yield but in many areas has been superceded by new ultrasound techniques such as cross-sectional and Doppler echocardiography.

References

1. Upton MT, Gibson DG: The study of left ventricular function from digitised echocardiograms. Prog Cardiovasc Dis 1978; 20: 359–384.
2. Upton MT, Gibson DG, Brown DJ: Echocardiographic assessment of abnormal left ventricular relaxation in man. British Heart Journal 1976; 38: 1001–1009.
3. Doran JH, Traill TA, Brown DJ, Gibson DG: Detection of abnormal wall movement during isovolumic contraction and early relaxation. Comparison of echo and angiocardiography. British Heart J 1974; 40: 361–71.
4. Traill TA, Gibson DG, Brown DJ: Study of left ventricular wall thickness and dimension changes using echocardiography. British Heart Journal 1978; 40: 162–169.
5. Hall RJC, Austin A, Hunter S: M-mode echogram as a means of distinguishing between mild and severe mitral stenosis. British Heart Journal 1980; 46: 486–491.
6. Furukawa K, Matsuura T, Endo N, Kunishige H, Tohara M, Watanabe T, Matsukubo H, Tsujii Y, Ijichi H: Use of digitised left ventricular echocardiograms in assessment of mitral stenosis. British Heart Journal 1978; 42: 176–181.
7. Bullock RE, Griffiths C, Amer H, Albers C, Appleton D, Hall RJC: Precision of digitised M-mode echocardiograms for clinical practice. European Heart J 1984; 5: 941–7.
8. Sutton MG.St.J, Traill TA, Ghafour AS, Brown DJ, Gibson DG: Echocardiographic assessment of left ventricular filling after mitral valve surgery. British Heart Journal 1977; 39: 1283–91.
9. Dawkins KD, Cotter L, Gibson DG: Assessment of mitral Bjork-Shiley prosthetic dysfunction using digitised M-mode echocardiography. British Heart Journal 1984; 51: 168–74.
10. Miller HC, Gibson DG, Stephens JD: Role of echocardiography and phonocardiography in diagnosis of mitral paraprosthetic regurgitation with Starr-Edwards prostheses. British Heart Journal 1973; 35: 1217–1225.
11. Venco A, St. John Sutton MG, Gibson DG, Brown DJ: Non-invasive assessment of left ventricular function after correction of severe aortic regurgitation. British Heart Journal 1976; 38: 1324–1331.
12. Gibson DG, Traill TA, Hall RJC, Brown DJ: Echocardiographic features of secondary left ventricular hypertrophy. British Heart Journal 1979; 41: 54–59.
13. Gibson DG, Prewitt TA, Brown DJ: Analysis of left ventricular wall movement during isovolumic relaxation and its relation to coronary artery disease. British Heart Journal 1976; 38: 1010–1019.

132

14. Hall RJC: M-mode echocardiography in the detection of surgically resectable left ventricular aneurysm. European Heart Journal, 1983; 4: 230–237.
15. Sutton MG.St.J, Reichek N, Kastor JA, Giuliani ER: Computerised M-mode echocardiographic analysis of left ventricular dysfunction in cardiac amyloid. Circulation 1982; 66: 790–799.

10. Reliability and Accuracy of Echocardiography for Follow-up Studies after Intervention

R. ERBEL, R. ZOTZ, B. HENKEL, G. SCHREINER, C. STEUERNAGEL, R. ZAHN, H. KOPP, W. CLAS, R. BRENNECKE, P. SCHWEIZER and J. MEYER
Johannes Gutenberg University, Mainz, FRG

By two-dimensional echocardiography limitations of M-mode echocardiography have been eliminated. As a direct and noninvasive method two-dimensional echocardiography seems to be an ideal method for analysis of left ventricular function in follow-up studies. In relation to other methods there are no limitations concerning x-ray exposure, physicians and patients safety. Before different studies can be discussed, reliability and accuracy of two-dimensional echocardiography have to be evaluated. Beat-to-beat, day-to-day, intra- and interobserver variability will be discussed, followed by description of follow-up studies after intervention.

Beat-to-beat variability

In 31 unselected patients 3 and 5 consecutive heart beats were evaluated and end-diastolic and end-systolic volume determined using a semi-automatic computer system by a disc method [1, 2]. Peak of the Q-wave was regarded as end-diastole, smallest ventricular silhouete as end-systole. Two-dimensional echocardiograms were recorded in the apical 4 chamber and RAO-equivalent view, using a Diasonics 3400 R real-time, phased array sector scanner. The 32-element 2.25 MHz transducer used has an active surface of 1.3×1.2 cm. The phased array principle enables an 84° sector to be visualized; a 15 cm depth was used. For statistical purposes mean values, standard deviations, factor loading, communalities and explained variance were analysed by a BMDP 4M-program of the Health Science computing faculty of the university of California, Los Angeles of 1979 [3]. Results of the statistical analysis for the RAO-equivalent view are listed in Table 1, demonstrating, that for end-diastolic and end-systolic volume values for explained variance were in the range of 95%. For the end-diastolic volume coefficient of variance was lower than for the endsystolic volume. For stroke volume and ejection fraction, explained variance measured 88% and 83%, respectively, with coefficients of variance of about 0.3 and 0.2. Correlation matrix showed very high values for the end-diastolic and end-systolic volume. As

J. Roelandt (editor), Digital Techniques in Echocardiography. ISBN 0-89838-861-9.

calculated parameters variance of end-diastolic and end-systolic volume is included in the reliability calculated for stroke volume and ejection fraction. Correlation coefficients were, thus, lower.

In comparison to the RAO-equivalent view, statistical analysis revealed a higher accuracy for the 4-chamber view. Explained variance for stroke volume and ejection fraction were 90% and 85% respectively. Coefficients of variance were below 0.3 for stroke volume and 0.2 for ejection fraction. Correlation matrix of 4-chamber view was in the same range as for the RAO-equivalent view (Table 2).

Analysis of 5 instead of 3 beats increased reliability for less than 1%. Particularly explained variance, which was high, could not be further increased. Thus, for calculation of end-diastolic and end-systolic volume as well as stroke volume

Table 1. Analysis of beat-to-beat variation for 3 consecutive cycles, using apical RAO-equivalent views (n = 24).

	End-diastolic volume				End-systolic volume		
	1st	2nd	3rd beat		1st	2nd	3rd beat
$\bar{X}$/ml	138	141	135		64	64	63
± S	44	41	47		34	32	35
Coefficient of variance	0.321	0.293	0.349		0.531	0.491	0.557
Communality	0.935	0.947	0.905		0.937	0.950	0.921
Factor loading	0.975	0.989	0.959		0.976	0.989	0.967
Explained variance		95%				96%	
Correlation matrix	EDV_1	EDV_2	EDV_3		ESV_1	ESV_2	ESV_3
EDV_1	1.000			ESV_1	1.000		
EDV_2	0.965	1.000		ESV_2	0.965	1.000	
EDV_3	0.935	0.948	1.000	ESV_3	0.904	0.956	1.000

	Stroke volume				Ejection fraction		
	1st	2nd	3rd beat		1st	2nd	3rd beat
$\bar{X}$/ml	74	77	72	$\bar{X}$%	55	56	55
± S	22	22	25	± S	11	11	12
Coefficient of variance	0.296	0.286	0.345		0.205	0.201	0.223
Communality	0.825	0.857	0.787		0.737	0.854	0.757
Factor loading	0.932	0.966	0.908		0.860	0.998	0.872
Explained variance		88%				83%	
Correlation matrix	SV_1	SV_2	SV_3		EF_1	EF_2	EF_3
SV_1	1.000			EF_1	1.000		
SV_2	0.900	1.000		EF_2	0.859	1.000	
SV_3	0.847	0.877	1.000	EF_3	0.750	0.870	1.000

and ejection fraction by two-dimensional echocardiography analysis of 3 consecutive heart beats is sufficient.

Radionuclide methods cannot be used for beat-to-beat analysis. Cineventriculography demonstrates no significant difference when two consecutive beats are evaluated [4]. Analysis of more beats is not possible cause of the negative inotropic effect of contrast agents [5, 6, 7].

Day-to-day variability

For analysis of day-to-day variability, 3 consecutive beats on three consecutive days were evaluated. Thus, it includes beat-to-beat and day-to-day variation.

Table 2. Analysis of beat-to-beat variation for 3 consecutive heart cycles, using apical 4-chamber views (n = 31).

	End-diastolic volume				End-systolic volume		
	1st	2nd	3rd beat		1st	2nd	3rd beat
$\bar{X}$/ml	156	162	155		86	92	85
$\pm$ S	53	56	49		48	52	46
Coefficient of variance	0.338	0.343	0.316		0.559	0.563	0.544
Communality	0.935	0.934	0.912		0.978	0.969	0.963
Factor loading	0.980	0.979	0.965		0.996	0.987	0.984
Explained variance		95%				98%	
Correlation matrix	EDV_1	EDV_2	EDV_3		ESV_1	ESV_2	ESV_3
EDV_1	1.000			ESV_1	1.000		
EDV_2	0.960	1.000		ESV_2	0.984	1.000	
EDV_3	0.946	0.945	1.000	ESV_3	0.980	0.972	1.000

	Stroke volume				Ejection fraction		
	1st	2nd	3rd beat		1st	2nd	3rd beat
$\bar{X}$/ml	68	68	65	$\bar{X}$%	54	57	54
$\pm$ S	20	19	16	$\pm$ S	10	10	9
Coefficient of variance	0.303	0.282	0.254		0.181	0.168	0.158
Communality	0.828	0.894	0.843		0.789	0.881	0.757
Factor loading	0.922	0.984	0.931		0.888	1.000	0.869
Explained variance		90%				85%	
Correlation matrix	SV_1	SV_2	SV_3		EF_1	EF_2	EF_3
SV_1	1.000			EF_1	1.000		
SV_2	0.907	1.000		EF_2	0.888	1.000	
SV_3	0.859	0.916	1.000	EF_3	0.751	0.869	1.000

Explained variance dropped for the RAO-equivalent view to 85% and 87% for end-diastolic and end-systolic volume (Table 3). For the 4-chamber view values were higher with 95% and 83% respectively (Table 4). Again, calculated parameters had lower explained variances and correlation coefficients (Table 4).

Mean difference for end-diastolic volume measured 5.5 ± 11.0 ml and for end-systolic volume 2.9 ± 12.5 ml, related to absolute values, standard deviation was $\pm 10.2\%$ and $\pm 13.6\%$ between the 1st and 2nd day and $\pm 8.9\%$ and $\pm 18.6\%$ between the 1st and 3rd day.

For stroke volume mean difference measured 0.6 ± 10.6 ml and for ejection fraction $1.5 \pm 11.7\%$. In relation to absolute values, standard deviation of the mean difference was $\pm 11.9\%$ and $\pm 19.7\%$ between 1st and 2nd day and $\pm 10.1\%$ and $\pm 11.7\%$ between 1st and 3rd day.

Table 3. Day-to-day variation for 3 consecutive days, using apical RAO-equivalent views (n = 16).

	End-diastolic volume				End-systolic volume		
	1st	2nd	3rd day		1st	2nd	3rd day
$\bar{X}$/ml	122	120	117		59	61	60
$\pm$ S	31	31	27		17	15	13
Coefficient of variance	0.256	0.255	0.232		0.283	0.240	0.214
Communality	0.942	0.945	0.900		0.583	0.906	0.924
Factor loading	0.982	0.985	0.956		0.757	0.951	1.000
Explained variance		95%				83%	
Correlation matrix	EDV_1	EDV_2	EDV_3		ESV_1	ESV_2	ESV_3
EDV_1	1.000			ESV_1	1.000		
EDV_2	0.967	1.000		ESV_2	0.689	1.000	
EDV_3	0.939	0.942	1.000	ESV_3	0.757	0.951	1.000

	Stroke volume				Ejection fraction		
	1st	2nd	3rd day		1st	2nd	3rd day
$\bar{X}$/ml	59	59	60	$\bar{X}$%	48	47	49
$\pm$ S	18	20	24	$\pm$ S	7	8	9
Coefficient of variance	0.300	0.346	0.400		0.133	0.168	0.175
Communality	0.789	0.865	0.891		0.666	0.706	0.663
Factor loading	0.902	0.946	0.980		0.868	0.907	0.866
Explained variance		79%				78%	
Correlation matrix	SV_1	SV_2	SV_3		EF_1	EF_2	EF_3
SV_1	1.000			EF_1	1.000		
SV_2	0.854	1.000		EF_2	0.787	1.000	
SV_3	0.884	0.927	1.000	EF_3	0.751	0.785	1.000

For cineventriculography only few publications can be analyzed. Cohn et al. [4] also found a higher variability for end-systolic than for end-diastolic volume in 5 patients. Mean difference for end-diastolic volume was 20 ml, for end-systolic volume 32 ml. Mean difference of ejection fraction was 19%. McAnulty et al. [8] published a mean difference of 6.2 ± 15.7% for this parameter. These results are in the range of our results for two-dimensional echocardiography.

For M-mode echocardiography a high reproducibility was described [9, 10, 11]. Stefadouros and Canedo [11] calculated a range for end-diastolic diameter from −3.5 to 3.5 mm and for end-systolic diameter from −2.5 to 2.5 mm. Percentage difference cannot be given cause of lack of absolute values. Pietro et al. [10] found a mean difference of 3.5% and 8.5% for end-diastolic and end-systolic diameter in follow-up studies. In a randomized placebo controlled study in patients with

Table 4. Day-to-day variation for 3 consecutive days, using apical 4-chamber views (n = 16).

	End-diastolic volume				End-systolic volume		
	1st	2nd	3rd day		1st	2nd	3rd day
$\bar{X}$/ml	115	118	121		52	51	54
± S	22	25	25		13	14	13
Coefficient of variance	0.192	0.208	0.201		0.253	0.270	0.236
Communality	0.880	0.889	0.659		0.827	0.907	0.800
Factor loading	0.957	0.979	0.824		0.908	1.000	0.893
Explained variance		85%				87%	
Correlation matrix	EDV_1	EDV_2	EDV_3		ESV_1	ESV_2	ESV_3
EDV_1	1.000			ESV_1	1.000		
EDV_2	0.936	1.000		ESV_2	0.908	1.000	
EDV_3	0.788	0.806	1.000	ESV_3	0.790	0.893	1.000

	Stroke volume				Ejection fraction		
	1st	2nd	3rd day		1st	2nd	3rd day
$\bar{X}$/ml	63	68	65	$\bar{X}$%	54	57	54
± S	19	19	19	± S	10	10	9
Coefficient of variance	0.303	0.282	0.254		0.181	0.168	0.158
Communality	0.828	0.894	0.843		0.789	0.881	0.757
Factor loading	0.922	0.984	0.931		0.888	1.000	0.869
Explained variance		90%				85%	
Correlation matrix	SV_1	SV_2	SV_3		EF_1	EF_2	EF_3
SV_1	1.000			EF_1	1.000		
SV_2	0.907	1.000		EF_2	0.888	1.000	
SV_3	0.859	0.916	1.000	EF_3	0.751	0.869	1.000

mitral valve prolapse syndrome mean difference between two measurements (4 weeks interval) was below 5% [12]. Martin and Fiedler [13] found a coefficient of variance of 3.4 for end-diastolic diameter and 8.4 for fractional shortening. Also for evaluated parameters in the placebo controlled study higher variability was found [12].

For radionuclide studies Wackers et al. [14] calculated in patients with normal left ventricular function a mean difference of 10% for ejection fraction and 5% in patients with heart disease. Thus, these authors regard in an individual patient a change of ejection fraction of 10% in patients with and 5% in patients with impaired left ventricular function as limits for assessing significant serial alterations in left ventricular ejection fraction in individual patients.

By two-dimensional echocardiography, in an individual patient a non random from a random change can be distinguished, when the change of end-diastolic volume is more than 10%, for the end-systolic volume more than 15%, for stroke volume more than 20% and for ejection fraction more than 10%.

Intraobserver variation

In 20 patients the same observer analyzed two-dimensional echocardiograms with a time interval of 4 to 6 weeks.

Percentage difference between both analysis was below 5% and standard deviation <10% (Table 5).

Whereas analysis of variance detected no significant difference between both analysis, the permutation test detected a significant difference for the end-diastolic volume (p <0.015) for the RAO equivalent view, but for the 4-chamber view no significant difference was found (Table 5). Again accuracy and reproducibility of the RAO equivalent view was lower than of the 4-chamber view.

Sigel et al. [15] observed a high reproducibility for cineventriculography. Correlation coefficients were 0.97 for end-diastolic, 0.14 for end-systolic volume and 0.95 for ejection fraction. Mean differences measured 0.4 ± 4.4 ml, 0.4 ± 8.0 ml and $0.4 \pm 2.4\%$ respectively. Chaitman et al. [16] found a mean difference of 4.8 ± 0.9 ml, 4.7 ± 1.4 ml and $2.1 \pm 0.3\%$.

For radionuclide studies Okada et al. [17] observed a mean intraobserver variation of 5.8% for ejection fraction. Wackers et al. [14] reported a mean difference of $1.4 \pm 1.2\%$ (0–5%) for the same parameter. As for the day-to-day variation, variability was higher in patients with normal than in patients with reduced left ventricular function. Similar results are reported for M-mode echocardiography by Pietro et al. [9]. ($5.8 \pm 18\%$ and $3.1 \pm 0.6\%$, respectively). Similar results are published by Lapido et al. [8].

Also other authors analyzed intraobserver variation of two-dimensional echocardiography. For left ventricular volume Touche et al. [18] measured a correlation coefficient of 0.986 and mean difference of 9 ml. Sold [19] found a mean difference of 12.1 (2.2–28.5) ml for end-diastolic, 7.8 (3.1–16.6) ml for end-systolic volume and 3.6 (0.8–7.2)% for ejection fraction, corresponding to a mean percentage difference of 11.1 (1.7–24.3)%, 14.1 (2.8–20.7)% and 6.0 (1.1–12.1)%, respectively. Compared to these results, our intraobserver variation is somewhat lower than those of Touche et al. [18], but better than that of Sold [19]. In relation to radionuclide studies results of intraobserver variation are comparable. Cause of the high resolution cineventriculography is superior to both noninvasive methods.

Interobserver variation

The two-dimensional echocardiographic studies were performed by the same technician and always 3 consecutive heart cycles were evaluated to receive the

Table 5. Intraobserver variability, tested in 20 patients with a time interval of 4–6 weeks. For statistical purposes Pitman test was used. Mean values ± standard deviation ($\bar{X} \pm S$), mean difference ± standard deviation ($\bar{D} \pm SD$), mean percentage difference ($\%\bar{D}$).

RAO	$\bar{X} \pm 33$	$\bar{D} \pm SD$	Range	$\%\bar{D}$	p
EDV_A/ml	126 ± 33				
		$3,8 \pm 7,3$	$+17,3/-10,3$	3,0	0.015
EDV_B/ml	122 ± 34				
ESV_A/ml	67 ± 28				
		$1,7 \pm 4,8$	$+11,7/-1.7$	2.5	0.064
ESV_B/ml	66 ± 29				
SV_A/ml	59 ± 17				
		$2,1 \pm 6.7$	$+17,0/-14,0$	3,6	0,098
SV_B/ml	57 ± 17				
EF_A/%	48 ± 12				
		0.1 ± 3.7	$+6,3/-10.4$	0,2	0,489
EF_B/%	48 ± 12				
4–C					
EDV_A/ml	125 ± 29				
		$1,2 \pm 6,7$	$+9,4/-12,4$	1,0	0,224
EDV_B/ml	126 ± 30				
ESV_A/ml	64 ± 24				
		$0,6 \pm 5,0$	$+11,0/-7,4$	1,0	0,294
ESV_B/ml	63 ± 25				
SV_A/ml	61 ± 18				
		$1,8 \pm 6,3$	$+8,3/-15.0$	3,0	0,115
SV_B/ml	63 ± 17				
EF_A/%	50 ± 11				
		1.2 ± 4.1	$+4,3/-11,0$	2,4	0,114
EF_B/%	51 ± 11				

maximum possible accuracy. Interobserver variability was analyzed by evaluation of two experienced observers. Permutation test revealed significant differences related to end-diastolic, end-systolic volume, as well as stroke volume, but not for ejection fraction using RAO equivalent view. Concerning the 4-chamber view no significant difference was detected (Table 6). The accuracy of different observers can be analyzed using calculation of the mean reliability and the smallest mean square difference. Thus, this method can be used before starting a study as a test for the reliability of the different observers.

Interobserver variation for cineventriculography tested by Cohn et al. [4] correlation coefficients measured 0.72, 0.87 and 0.83 for end-diastolic, end-systolic volume and ejection fraction. Mean difference for these parameters were 20 ml, 10 ml and 5%, in the same range as results for two-dimensional echocardiography. Previous reports, however, presented a much better interobserver variability [15, 16, 20]. The improved technique of x-ray systems seems to be a

Table 6. Interobserver variability (1/2) tested in 20 patients. For statistical purposes Pitman test was used. Mean values ± standard deviation ($\bar{X} \pm S$), mean difference ± standard deviation ($\bar{D} \pm SD$), mean percentage difference ($\bar{D}\%$).

RAO	$\bar{X} \pm S$	$\bar{D} \pm SD$	$\bar{D}\%$	P
EDV_1/ml	126 ± 33			
		12.3 ± 14.4	9.8	0.001
EDV_2/ml	138 ± 39			
ESV_1/ml	67 ± 28			
		5.7 ± 15.9	8.5	0.07
ESV_2/ml	73 ± 23			
SV_1/ml	59 ± 17			
		6.7 ± 18.6	11.4	0.06
SV_2/ml	65 ± 22			
EF_1/%	48 ± 12			
		0.9 ± 12.2	1.9	0.38
EF_2/%	47 ± 8			
4–C				
EDV_1/ml	125 ± 29			
		5.4 ± 17.6	4.3	0.093
EDV_2/ml	130 ± 35			
ESV_1/ml	64 ± 24			
		3.7 ± 14.7	5.8	0.140
ESV_2/ml	68 ± 22			
SV_1/ml	61 ± 18			
		1.8 ± 14.1	2.9	0.295
SV_2/ml	62 ± 16			
EF_1/%	50 ± 11			
		1.0 ± 8.2	2.0	0.794
EF_2/%	49 ± 6			

141

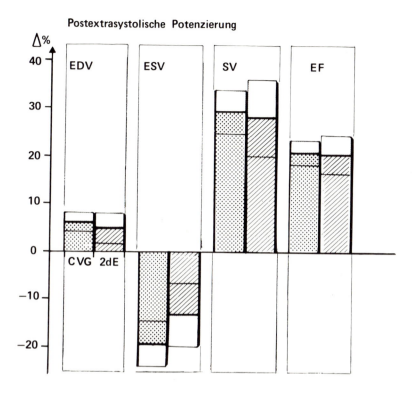

Fig. 1. Percentage changes of end-diastolic and end-systolic volume (EDV/ESV), stroke volume (SV), and ejection fraction (EF) for two-dimensional echocardiography (2dE) and cineventriculography (CVG) after postextrasystolic potention. $\bar{X} \pm SD$.

possible explanation. Radionuclide studies reported a mean difference for ejection fraction of $1.6 \pm 1.5\%$ (0–6%) [14], 6.0% [21] and 6% [17]. Mean difference for ejection fraction in our studies was $1.0 \pm 8.2\%$.

In comparison to two-dimensional echocardiography, M-mode echocardiography has a higher reproducibility and lower and not significant interobserver variability [9]. In future improvement of resolution of two-dimensional echocardiography will lead to lower interobserver variation. Concerning ejection fraction, however, no significant difference between different experienced observers have to be expected.

Intervention studies

The accuracy of echocardiography in intervention studies – the prediction before the method can be used for pharmacodynamic studies – was tested in comparison to cineventriculography for (1) postextrasystolic potentiation, (2) effect of positive inotropic agents, (3) effect of thrombolysis therapy, and (4) effect of an-

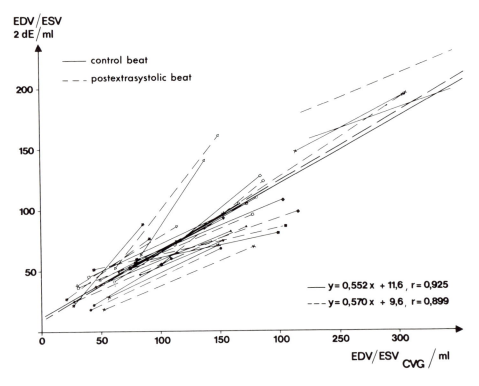

Fig. 2. Illustration of the end-diastolic (EDV) and end-systolic (ESV) volume for different patients before (——) and after (– – – –) postextrasystolic potentiation. Correlation coefficients and regression equation are given.

gioplasty. Changes after postextrasystolic potentiation and injection of prenalterol were evaluated by simultaneous analysis of cineventericulography and echocardiography. During cineventriculography in the RAO projection, apical two-dimensional echocardiograms were recorded in the RAO-equivalent view. Thus, radiographic contrast injection was used as echocardiographic contrast, too [22].

(1) Postextrasystolic potentiation

The positive inotropic effect of postextrasystolic potentiation increased stroke volume and ejection fraction significantly (Figure 1). End-diastolic volume increased for +5.9% and +4.8%, respectively, whereas end-systolic volume decreased for +19.3% and 19.7%. Increase of stroke volume measured 29.2 and 28.1%. Mehmel et al. [23] reported an increase of ejection fraction from 43 to 57%, Azancot et al. [24] from 42% to 57%. Similar changes were observed in our study. For cineventriculography ejection fraction increased from 55% to 66%

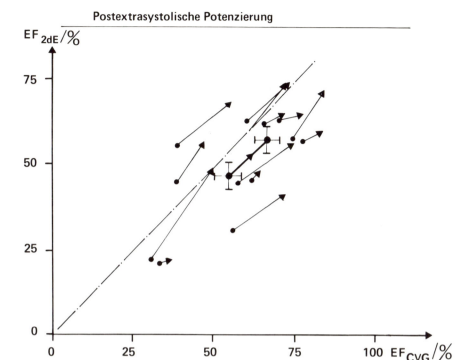

Fig. 3. Comparison between left ventricular ejection fraction determined echocardiographically and cineventriculographically (2DE/CVG) for control (●) and postextrasystolic potentiation (▲). Regression equation for control was y = 0.737x + 12.8, r = 0.787 and postextrasystolic beats y = 0.735x + 17.2, r = 0.835. It can be seen, that the changes observed were parallel to the regression line of the control beat.

and two-dimensional echocardiography from 47% to 57%. Percentage change amounted to 20.9% and 20.7%. Despite differences in absolute values, percentage changes were comparable for stroke volume and ejection fraction. These results are based on the observation, that the change of left ventricular function did not alter the relation between both methods for end-diastolic and end-systolic volume. In Figure 2 is illustrated, that only a parallel shift of the relation between both parameters is found. Thus, regression equation remained nearly unchanged: Y = 0.552 × + 11.6, r = 0.925, and Y = 0.570 × + 9.6, r = 0.899 respectively. Similar changes were observed for ejection fraction (Figure 3).

(2) Positive inotropic agents (Prenalterol)

Compared to postextrasystolic potentiation end-diastolic and end-systolic volume decreased after injection of prenalterol [25, 26]. Drop of end-diastolic volume measured 5% and 8% for cineventriculography and two-dimensional

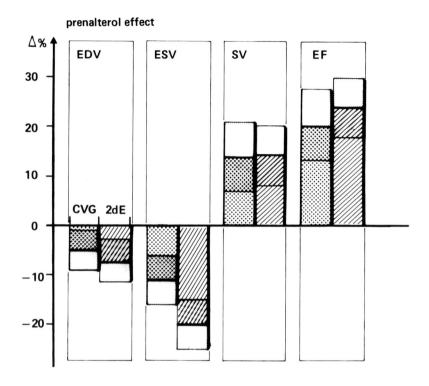

prenalterol effect

Δ%

EDV   ESV   SV   EF

CVG 2dE

Fig. 4. Percentage change of end-diastolic and end-systolic volume (EDV/ESV), stroke volume (SV) and ejection fraction (EF) after intravenous application of prenalterol for two-dimensional echocardiography (2dE) and cineventriculography (CVG). X̄ ± SD.

echocardiography and end-systolic volume 12% and 21%. In 4 patients even an increase of end-diastolic volume was observed determined by cineventriculography, in 3/4 patients also found by two-dimensional echocardiography. Also, Greene et al. [27] reported an increase of end-diastolic volume by cineventriculography in patients with severe impaired left ventricular function related to an increase in compliance and relaxation. Change of ejection fraction measured 5.6% and 8.4%, of stroke volume 10.5 and 11.6 ml, respectively. Measured range for two-dimensional echocardiographic and cineventriculographic changes of stroke volume and ejection fraction, again, were in the same range despite differences in absolute values. An increase of 20 and 22% respectively was observed (Figure 4). In the correlation between both methods, a slight parallel shift of the regression line is observed. Only one patient showed a non parallel shift (Figure 5). Regression coefficients, y-axis intercept as well as correlation coefficients remained nearly unchanged.

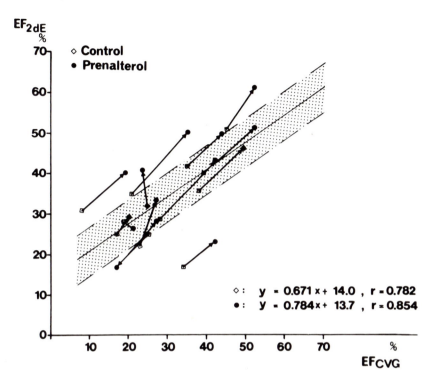

Fig. 5. Correlation of the left ventricular ejection fraction determined by two-dimensional echocardiography (2dE) and cineventriculography (CVG) before ▣ and after ● administration of prenalterol. It can be seen, that the changes occur in parallel to the regression equation of the study before administration of the drug.

(3) Thrombolysis therapy

To be as quick as possible in restoration of coronary blood flow in acute myocardial infarction cineventriculography was not performed prior to coronary angiography. Here, two-dimensional echocardiography offers the possibility of evaluation of left ventricular function and wall motion prior to thrombolysis therapy during preparation of cardiac catheterization.

We compared the effect of thrombolysis therapy in patients with and without angioplasty as well as with anterior and inferior myocardial infarction. Cineventriculograms were performed after the end of intracoronary thrombolysis and angioplasty, as described previously [27]. Within 15 min, also apical two-dimensional echocardiograms were recorded. Control studies were performed 4 weeks later before discharge. In Figure 6, change of end-diastolic and end-systolic volume index as well as stroke volume index and ejection fraction is demonstrated after thrombolysis with (I) and without (II) angioplasty. It can be seen, than in patients with PTCA a higher increase of ejection fraction could be

146

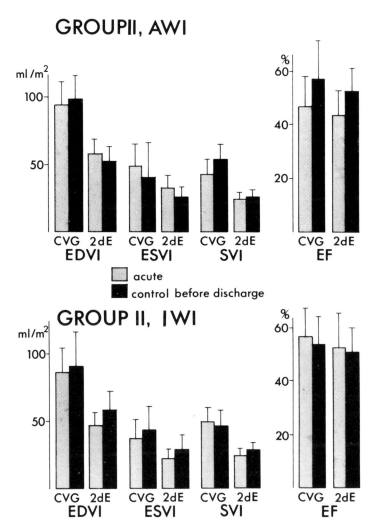

Fig. 6. End-diastolic and end-systolic volume index (EDVI/ESVI), stroke volume index (SVI) and ejection fraction (EF) in patients with thrombolysis therapy measured by two-dimensional echocardiography (2dE) and cineventriculography (CVG). It is obvious, that the direction and the amount of change for all parameters are comparable for both methods.

observed in comparison to patients without angioplasty. The change from the acute to the control study before discharge revealed same direction for two-dimensional echocardiography as cineventriculography.

Despite significant differences in absolute values for end-diastolic and end-systolic volume percentage change for the most important diameters stroke volume and ejection fraction were in the same range. That means, that two-dimensional echocardiography can be regarded as an accurate method for analysis of left ventricular function particularly suitable in patients with thrombolysis

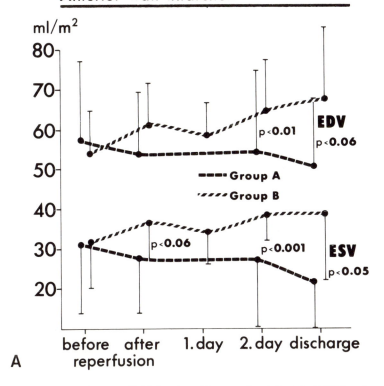

Fig. 7a. Acute transmural myocardial infarction. Changes of end-diastolic (EDV) and end-systolic volume (ESV) as well as ejection fraction (EF) in patients with PTCA after thrombolysis therapy.

7 a: Changes of end-diastolic and end-systolic volume (EDV/ESV) index.

7 b: Changes of ejection fraction.

Indicated are values for acute and control before discharge analyzed by two-dimensional echocardiography (2dE). $\bar{X} \pm SD$.

Group A: infarct time <3 h 30 min; group B: in farct time >3 h 30 min.

therapy where in follow-up studies this noninvasive method is needed. In Figure 7 changes of left ventricular volumes and ejection fraction is demonstrated in patients with infarct times – time between onset of symptoms and restoration of coronary blood flow – of more and less than 3 h 30 min. It can be seen that in patients with short infarct times ejection fraction improves immediately after thrombolysis therapy, and is even after 4 weeks higher than in patients with long infarct times [28].

(4) Coronary angioplasty (PTCA)

During angioplasty, severe myocardial ischemia developes because of the interrupted blood flow except in patients with collaterals.

148

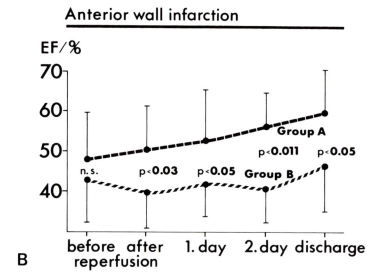

Fig. 7b. Changes of left ventricular ejection fraction in patients with time between onset of symptoms until reperfusion of <3 h 30 min (Group A) and >3 h 30 min (Group B) $\bar{X} \pm SD$).

We studied the effect of PTCA on left ventricular function by two-dimensional echocardiography using the apical approach. During angioplasty end-diastolic volume is slightly, but end-systolic volume significantly increased. Ejection fraction decreased cause of reduced regional wall motion induced by PTCA (Figure 8). These observed changes of left ventricular function started well before ST-segment changes and angina pectoris.

In consecutive dilations, changes of left ventricular function are similar. Here is demonstrated that the reproducibility of two-dimensional echocardiography for intervention studies is very high. End-diastolic volume and end-systolic volume are significantly reduced after intracoronary injection of nitroglycerine. Wall stress and oxygen demand is reduced. Drop of left ventricular ejection fraction during dilation is smaller after administration of nitroglycerine. The most significant effect is observed one minute after intracoronary injection. After 5 and 10 minutes nitroglycerine effect decreased. Dilation time can, thus, be increased as a sign of increased ischemic tolerance [29, 30]. When nifedipine is injected, no significant change on left ventricular function during consecutive dilations could be observed as the drug has no effect on preload. Particularly end-diastolic and end-systolic volume remained constant. Control studies after 5 and 10 minutes showed comparable results (Figure 10)..

149

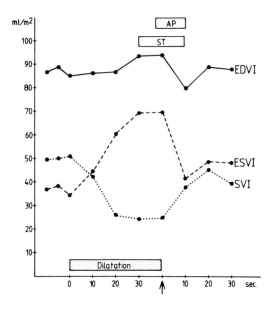

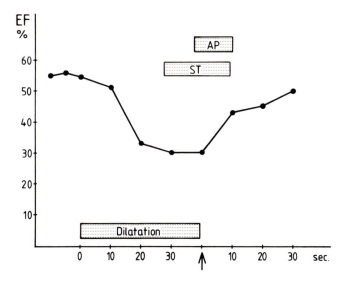

Fig. 8. Analysis of left ventricular function (end-diastolic, end-systolic and stroke volume as well as ejection fraction) during coronary angioplasty by apical two-dimensional echocardiography using RAO-equivalent view in a patient with dilation of left anterior descending coronary artery. Indicated are also the period of angina pectoris (AP) and time of appearance and disappearance of ST segment changes (ST).

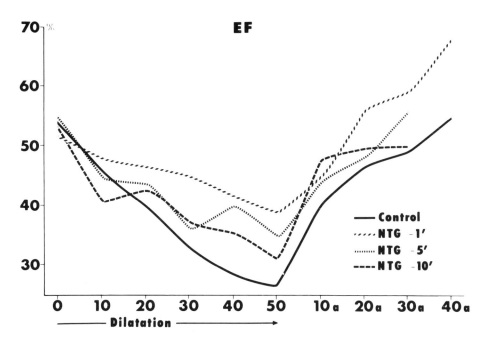

Fig. 9. Follow-up of left ventricular ejection fraction during coronary angioplasty before 1, 5, 10 min after intracoronary application of 0,2 mg nitroglycerine.

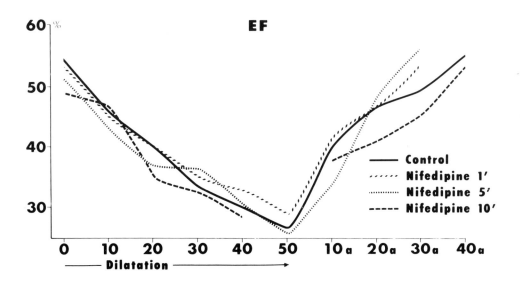

Fig. 10. Follow-up of left ventricular ejection during coronary angioplasty before 1, 5, 10 min after intracoronary administration of 0,2 mg nifedipine.

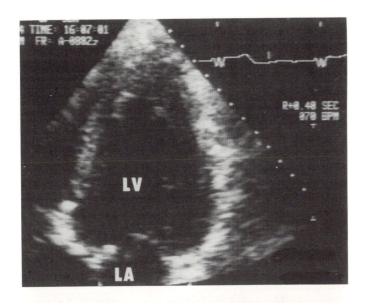

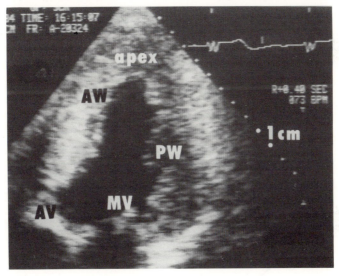

Fig. 11. Demonstration of enhancement of myocardial imaging after injection of 1 ml gelifundol into the aortic root in a patient with aortic stenosis. Illustrated is the improved possibility of endocardial border delineation of the left ventricle (LV). AW = anterior wall, PW = posterior wall, MV = mitral valve, AV = aortic valve, LA = left atrium.

6. Contrast echocardiography

The main problem for echocardiography is to receive good and high quality studies. Particularly endocardial border delineation is a crucial point. Using automatic computer analysis and digital subtraction echocardiography reproducibility can be improved as Grube et al. [31] pointed out. In patients with reduced left ventricular function, adverse reaction on contrast material, renal insufficiency as well as severe valvular heart disease left ventricular echoventriculography instead of cineventriculography can be used. But we also inject contrast material (Gelifundol° – a gelatine solution) in the aortic root. Reflection of left ventricular myocardium is enhanced (Figure 11) and better delineation of endocardial border is possible. Figure 11 demonstrates the increase of endocardial border delineation. Analysis of left ventricular volume and ejection fraction in these patients in comparison to cineventriculography revealed, that using this method ejection fraction could be determined in the same range as by cineventriculography. Determination of left ventricular parameters by apical two-dimensional echocardiography by an improved accuracy is related to a better delineation of left ventricular end-systolic contour (Table 7).

Conclusion

Two-dimensional echocardiography can be used for follow-up studies after intervention when echocardiograms of high quality are used and limitations of the method are known. Standardization should be as high as possible. Accuracy of two-dimensional echocardiography will be increased in the near future using digital imaging techniques and left side contrast echocardiography using myocardial perfusion phase for better delineation of endocardial contour.

Table 7. Analysis of end-diastolic and end-systolic volume (EDV/ESV) and left ventricular ejection fraction (EF) by apical two-dimensional echocardiography using the RAO-equivalent view. The mean of 3 consecutive heart beats are determined for images without (A) and with injection of gelifundol (B), after enhancement of myocardial reflection (C), after aortic root injection and for cineventriculography (CVG). Demonstrated is the improved accuracy of two-dimensional echocardiography by enhancement of myocardial imaging.

	2dE			CVG
	A	B	C	
EDV/ml	267	284	217	241
ESV/ml	145	165	112	115
EF/%	45	43	51	51

References

1. Erbel R, Krebs W, Henn G, Schweizer P, Richter HA, Meyer J, Effert S: Comparison of single-plane and biplane volume determination by two-dimensional echocardiography. I. Asymmetric model hearts. Eu Heart J 1982; 3: 469–480.

2. Erbel R, Schweizer P, Meyer J, Krebs W, Yalkinoglu Ö, Effert S: Sensitivity of cross-sectional echocardiography in detection of impaired global and regional left ventricular function: prospective study. Int J Cardiol 1985; 7: 375–389.

3. Erbel R: Funktionsdiagnostik des linken Ventrikels mittels zweidimensionaler Echokardiographie. Steinkopff Verlag Darmstadt, 1983.

4. Cohn P, Levine JA, Bergeron A, Gorlin R: Reproducibility of the angiography left ventricular ejection fraction in patients with coronary artery disease. Am Heart J 1984; 88: 713–720.

5. Carleton RA: Change in left ventricular volume during angiocardiography. Am J Cardiol 1971; 27: 60–463.

6. Erbel R, Neuhaus KL, Spiller P, Benn M, Kreuzer H: Beeinflussung der systolischen und diastolischen Ventrikelfunktion durch Kontrastmittelinjection in den linken Ventrikel. Z Kardiol 1976; 65: 305–318.

7. Vine DL, Hegg TD, Dodge HT, Stewart DK, Frimer M: Immediate effect of contrast medium injection on left ventricular volumes and ejection fraction – a study using metallic epicardial markers. Circulation 1977; 56: 379–384.

8. McAnulty JH, Kremkau EL, Rosch J, Hattenhauer MT, Rahimtoola SH: Spontaneous changes in left ventricular function between sequential studies. Am J Cardiol 1974; 34: 23–28.

9. Lapido GOA, Dunn FG, Pringle TH, Bastian B, Lawrie TDV: Serial measurements of left ventricular dimensions by echocardiography. Assessment of weak-to-weak, inter- and intra-observer variability in normal subjects and patients with valvular heart disease. Br Heart J 1980; 44: 284–289.

10. Pietro DA, Voelkel AG, Ray BJ, Parisi AF: Reproducibility of echocardiography. A study evaluating the variability of serial echocardiographic measurements. Chest 1981; 79: 29–32.

11. Stefadouros MA, Canedo MJ: Reproducibility of echocardiographic estimates of left ventricular dimensions. Br Heart J 1977; 39: 390–398.

12. Erbel R, Schweizer P, Merx W, Effert S: Kontrollierte Langzeitbehandlung des Mitralklappenprolapssyndroms mit Propranolol. Z Kardiol 1978; 67: 729–735.

13. Martin MA, Fiedler NRJ: Echocardiography in cardiovascular drug assessment. Br Heart J 1979; 41: 536–543.

14. Wackers FJT, Berger HJ, Johnstone DE, Goldman L, Reduto A, Langou RA, Gottschalk B, Zaret L: Multiple gated cardiac blood pool imaging for left ventricular ejection fraction, validation of the technique and assessment of variability. Am J Cardiol 1979; 43: 1159–1166.

15. Sigel H, Nechwatal W, Stauch M: Zur Frage der Reproduzierbarkeit von Parameern der quantitativen globalen und regionalen Lävangiographie im intra- und interindividuellen Observer-Vergleich. Z Kardiol 1981; 70: 742–747.

16. Chaitman BR, DeMots H, Bristow JD, Rösch J, Rahimtoola SH: Objective and subjective analysis of left ventricular angiograms. Circulation 1975; 52: 420–425.

17. Okada RD, Kirshenbaum HD. Kushner FG, Strauss W, Dinsmore RE, Newell JB, Boucher CA, Block PC, Pohost GM: Observer variance in the qualitative evaluation of left ventricular wall motion and quantitation of left ventricular ejection fraction using rest and exercise multigated blood pool imaging. Circulation 1980; 61: 128–136.

18. Touche T, Prasquier R, Merillon JP, Barthelemy M, Hanoun HC, Vervin P, Gourgon R: Mesure des volumes ventriculaires gauches par echographic bidimensinelle a partir d'une coupe apicale. Arch Med Coeur 1980; 73: 691–700.

19. Sold G, Kreuzer H: Erlaubt die zweidimensionale Echokardiographie eine verläßliche Bestimmung linksventrikulärer Funktionsgrößen? Kontroverse Ansichten in der Echokardiographie.

154

Hrsg G Biamino, L Lange, Schattauer, Stuttgart, 1984, p 265–275.

20. Rogers WJ, Bream PR, Smith LR, Williams SE, Rackley CE, Russell Jr RO: Effect if filming projection and interobserver variability on angiographic biplane left ventricular volume determination. Circulation 1979; 59: 96–104.

21. Greene DG, Carlisle R, Grant C, Brunnell L: Estimation of left ventricular volume by one-plane cineangiography. Circulation 1967; 35: 61–69.

22. Erbel R, Schweizer P, Lambertz H, Henn G, Meyer J, Krebs W, Effert S: Echoventriculography-A simultaneous analysis of two-dimensional echocardiography and cineventriculography. Circulation 1984; 67: 205–215.

23. Mehmel HC, Katus H, Bassemir KR, von Olshausen K, Zebe H, Kübler W: Comparison between the effect of postextrasystolic potentiation and the effect of nitrates on the left ventricular function for the differentiation between reversible and irreversible left ventricular asynergy. Basic Res Cardiol 1980; 75: 390–399.

24. Azancot J, Beaufils P, Masquet C, Georgiopoulos G, Dabalis D, Lorente P, Baudouy Y, Slama R, Bouvrain Y: Detection of residual myocardial function in acute transmural infarction using postextrasystolic potentiation. Circulation 1981; 64: 46–53.

25. Erbel R, Schweizer P, Lambertz H, Voelker W, Meyer J, Effert S: Echoventricular analysis of prenalterol induced changes of left ventricular function. Circulation 1981; 64 Suppl A: 49.

26. Erbel R, Meyer J, Lambertz H, Schweizer P, Voelker W, Krebs W, Braun G, Effert S: Hemodynamic effects of prenalterol in patients with ischemic heart disease and congestive cardiomyopathy. Circulation 1982; 66: 361–369.

27. Erbel R, Pop T, Meinertz Th, Kasper W, Schreiner G, Henkel B, Henrich KJ, Pfeiffer C, Rupprecht HJ, Meyer J: Combined medical and mechanical recanalization in acute myocardial infarction. Cath Cardiovasc Diagn 1985; 11: 361–377.

28. Erbel R, Pop T, Meinertz T, Clas W, Henkel B, Schreiner G, Steuernagel C, Meyer J: Analysis of left ventricular function before and immediately after recnalaization in acute myocardial infarction. Europ Heart J 1984; 5 Suppl 1: 220.

29. Erbel R, Schreiner G, Henkel B, Pop T, Meyer J: Improved ischemic tolerance during percutaneous transluminal coronary angioplasty by intracoronary injection of nitroglycerine. Z Kardiol 1983; 72 Suppl 3: 71–73.

30. Schreiner G, Erbel R, Henkel B, Pop T, Meyer J: Improved ischemic tolerance during percutaneous coronary angioplasty (PTCA) by antianginal drugs. Europ Heart J 1984; 5 Suppl I: 93.

31. Grube E: Automatic contour detection and subtraction technique for analysis of left ventricular function. In: Digital Techniques in Echocardiography, ed J Roelandt, Martinus Nijhoff, Dordrecht (in press).

11. Real-time, Orthogonal Cardiac Imaging*

JOSEPH KISSLO, JONATHAN E. SNYDER and OLAF T. VON RAMM
Duke University, Durham, North Carolina, USA

Introduction

Heart diseases result in changes in the thickness of heart walls and valves as well as in alterations in the size and shape of the heart chambers [1]. In order to visualize these changes, Edler and Hertz [2] utilized ultrasound as a unique method for providing spatial anatomic information. First M-mode, then two-dimensional echocardiography, came into common clinical use for evaluating cardiac disorders [3–8].

Full appreciation of the spatial geometry of the heart still depends upon a series of one or two-dimensional sonic interrogations requiring the interpreter to mentally reconstruct the heart in three dimensions. Three-dimensional echocardiographic methods developed to date require offline processing, frequently using a computer [9–13]. In order to implement a real-time multiplane imaging system, two technical barriers must be overcome. First, a transducer of sufficiently small size capable of multiplane imaging from within an intercostal space must be developed. Second, B-mode instrumentation must be improved to facilitate the high data acquisition rates necessary for real-time multiplane interrogations.

This manuscript presents the results from a new ultrasound imaging modality which permits high data acquisition rates and, by utilizing a novel transducer, the acquisition of two orthogonal planes (O-mode) in real-time. The present developmental work was undertaken on the hypothesis that construction of such a system could be realized.

Methods

Patients: O-mode examinations were performed on 50 consecutive patients undergoing clinical echocardiographic examination for a variety of reasons. There were 27 males and 33 females, aging in range from 29 to 78 years (mean 52 years).

*Supported in part by USPHS Grants HL-12715, CA-37586 and HL-07063 Bethesda, Maryland, USA

J. Roelandt (editor), Digital Techniques in Echocardiography. ISBN 0-89838-861-9.

156

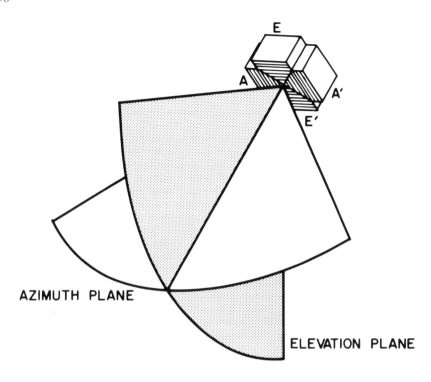

Fig. 1. Schematic of the bow-tie transducer and orientation of the orthogonal sector arcs. Four separate, nearly triangular, sections (A, A′, E, and E′) comprise the O-mode array.

Transducer: The O-mode transducer illustrated in Figure 1 is composed of two modified bow-tie shaped linear arrays assembled to form a cross. The array consists of four roughly triangular sections of piezoelectric ceramic, each cut into 16 elements and operates at 2.5 MHz. The finished transducer is mounted in a hand held case shown in Figure 2 and consists of two perpendicular linear arrays, each with a 20 mm aperture containing 32 elements. At the site of skin contact the transducer measures 22 × 22 mm.

System operation: O-mode has been implemented on both the original Duke University phased array ultrasound scanner [6,7] and the new version of this system. The current machine is a 32 transmit, 32 receive channel device with independent control over a 10 microsecond delay envelope of all channels. Analog receive processing is employed and the scanner has an operational bandwidth in excess of 5 MHz. This research device allows considerable freedom in the selection of imaging parameters by using a PDP 11/40 digital computer which executes the machine control software and provides editing facilities for O-mode software modifications.

In order to use the full 32 channels of the B-mode system in each plane and to avoid the cost and complexity of using two individual scanning systems, a tech-

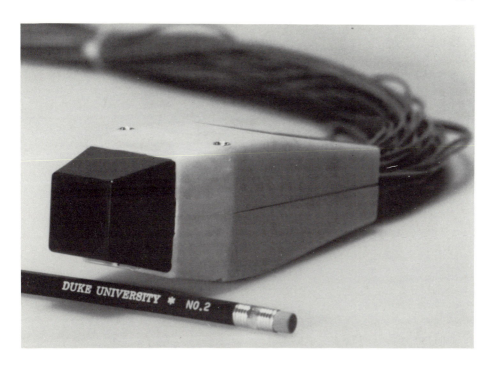

Fig. 2. The O-mode array is mounted in a hand held case.

nique for switching the available transmit and receive channels between the arrays was developed. Computer controlled receive multiplexers were constructed to rapidly switch the scanner's receive channels between the two linear arrays, permitting 'simultaneous' biplane scanning.

Each array aperture generates its own pie-shaped sector arc composed of 160 B-mode lines with an azimuth angle of 70°. The scan planes are orthogonal as seen in Figure 1, and contain unique anatomic information, except for the image line where the planes intersect, known as the boresight.

In the current implementation, O-mode images are displayed simultaneously in two sector arcs at a rate of 15 images per second. The frame rate is limited by the velocity of sound in tissue (1540 meters per second), making it impossible to acquire conventionally the complete image data in less than 1/15th of a second. By employing a parallel receive processing system referred to as Explososcan [14], it is possible to increase the data acquisition rate by a factor of four, facilitating an image rate of 60 frames per second. This four fold increase in frame rate is achieved by generating four receive image lines for each transmit pulse.

Figure 3 is a block diagram of the O-mode system, showing the additional processing circuitry, the Receive Multiplexer and Parallel Receive Processor, required for O-mode operation in conjunction with the phased array scanner. It utilizes two 32 element bow-tie arrays operating at a center frequency of 2.5

158

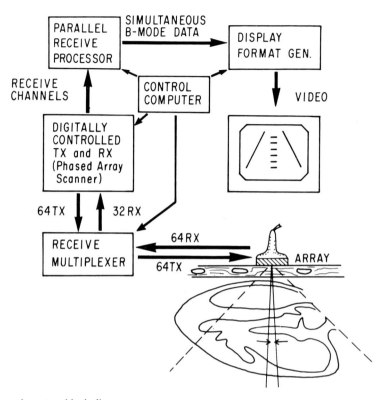

Fig. 3. O-mode system block diagram.

MHz. Image formation, controlled by the computer, begins with the creation of a B-mode line in one sector arc. The system then switches to the orthogonal sector to create the next line. This process is repeated until the full O-mode image is created.

The first O-mode prototype utilized the original Duke phased array scanner with Explososcan [15] to present the two 160 line orthogonal sectors simultaneously at a rate of 60 images per second. Results presented here were obtained with an improved array configuration on the new Duke system for which Explososcan is currently being modified. When the system is complete, O-mode will display 160 lines of B-mode data in each sector (total 320 lines) at a range of 13 cm and a rate of 60 frames per second. Conventional commercially available scanners do not have a comparable data acquisition rate and cannot obtain the acoustic data as rapidly.

Display: Figure 4 is an illustration of two of the O-mode display techniques. Figure 4A shows the bisection of a cylinder with two intersecting orthogonal planes. A simple method for the simultaneous display of two images is to position the conventional sector arcs side by side on a single display monitor as in Figure

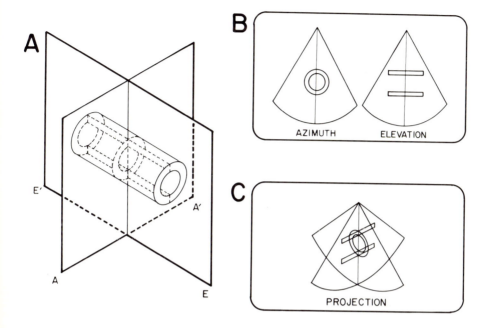

Fig. 4. Schematic diagram showing the intersection of two orthogonal planes (A-A′ and E-E′) with a circular cylinder (Panel A). The resulting sector arcs may be displayed side by side (Panel B) where the short and long axes of the cylinder are shown. The scan planes may be displayed in projection, individually or simultaneously (Panel C), to convey the three-dimensional nature of the image data.

4B. Unfortunately, this technique does not portray the three-dimensional nature of the image data. The spatial relationship between the planes is easier to convey by displaying simultaneously the two-dimensional projection of the two orthogonal sector arcs as indicated in Figure 4C. This method was implemented by modifying the software controlling the display monitor [16]. Under the current O-mode software, the user is able to select from three display modalities: side by side, single plane projection, and simultaneous projections. Although the axial rotations for the projection display are altered easily, a 45° rotation about the boresight for each of the two sectors and a 30° rotation about the axis parallel to the display screen (toward the observer) provide the most useful three-dimensional perspective without distorting the image.

Results

Beam profiles: The transducer shape does introduce an amplitude apodization across the aperture, altering its imaging characteristics from those of a normal rectangular array. *In vitro* azimuthal beam response plots shown in Figure 5 were obtained to quantify and compare the performance of the O-mode array (solid

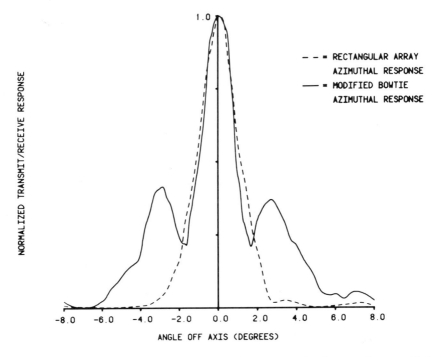

Fig. 5. Diagrammatic azimuthal (lateral) beam plots from a conventional rectangular array (dashed line) and from the O-mode bowtie array (solid line). The 'humps' on the sides of the solid line represent the sidelobes in the bowtie array. For details, see text.

line) with a normal transducer (dashed line). The beam response at the focal point for a normal 20 mm aperture array has a −6dB beam width of 1.2°. The O-mode response at the focal point has a −6dB beam width of 0.9°, but the signal-to-sidelobe ratio has been decreased by 27 dB. As determined with an AIUM standard test object, the normal system has a resolution of 1.5 mm in range and 2 mm in azimuth. The O-mode range resolution is equivalent, but the azimuthal resolution is reduced to 3 mm. This means that the effective resolution of the O-mode system is less than that of the normal scanner and additional artifact is noted in the images due to increased sidelobe levels.

Clinical images: It should be recognized that images from the new Duke University research prototype system are different from those seen on current commercial phased array devices. This machine uses an analog scan conversion format where the image is displayed on a monitor and recorded onto video tape via a television camera aimed at the display. This technique results in display processing that is different from that used in digital scan conversion systems. Scan lines are present in the images and target information appears to be less discrete in comparison to commercial scanners.

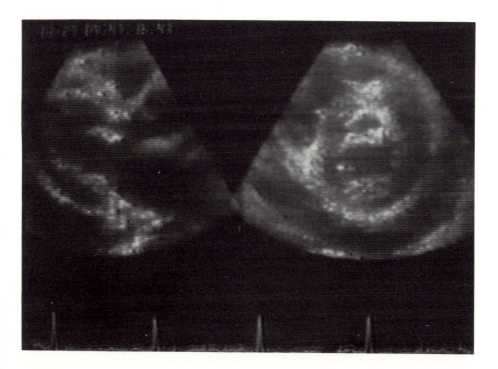

Fig. 6. Side by side simultaneous sector arcs showing the long axis (left side) and short axis (right side) of the left ventricle. Note the large pericardial effusion.

Scanning of the heart is conducted similarly to routine two-dimensional scanning beginning with the long axis of the left ventricle. O-mode is then switched on and the orthogonal view of the ventricular short axis is simultaneously presented side by side with the long axis as illustrated in Figure 6. The operator may then select the single sector projection (Figure 7A and 7B), or simultaneously (Figure 7C). Note that the simultaneous projection images contain a large quantity of data, requiring the user to become accustomed to this format. In these series of illustrations the long axis intersects with the short axis at the level of the papillary muscles.

At initial inspection, even the most experienced echo-cardiographer may think that the side-by-side images in Figure 6 are different than the projected images in Figure 7. Despite minor differences in transducer angulation, both sets of images have the same line densities and frame rates. The perceived differences are the optical result of the projection technique requiring the line densities of the scan planes shown in Figure 7 to appear non uniform; more dense in the foreground and less dense on the far edges of the sector arcs. Thus, although the acoustic data is the same in the two presentation formats, visual differences are perceived.

The ability to obtain information from the moving images on line, or from a video tape playback, is clearly superior to when the images are presented in still

162

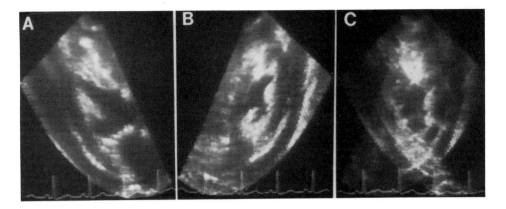

Fig. 7. Single plane projections in the long axis (Panel A) and short axis (Panel B) of the left ventricle from the same patient shown in Figure 6. The intersecting images are at the mid papillary level (Panel C). Note the perception of depth conveyed by these projections.

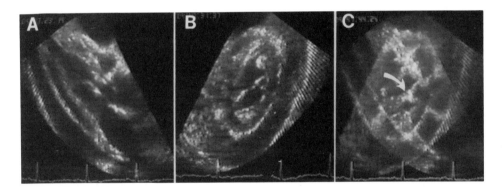

Fig. 8. Single plane projections in the long axis (Panel A) and short axis (Panel B) of the left ventricle from another patient with pericardial effusion. Simultaneous projections of the two sector arcs show the criss-cross pattern (Panel C, arrow) of the anterior mitral valve leaflet. Targets seen in both planes create a crossing pattern at the boresight.

frame. Still frames of these intersecting projected planes are particularly confusing since targets are superimposed and no movement is available to assist the observer in differentiating the planes. Structures imaged in both planes are identified by a crossing pattern seen at the boresight. The cross created by the presence of the anterior mitral valve leaflet in Figure 8 (Panel C, arrow) is one of the visual cues conveying the orthogonality of the sectors.

Because of the slight reduction in resolution and increased sidelobe levels with O-mode, the best quality scans are made with the gain reduced, thus enhancing resolution and reducing overall image noise.

Discussion

Previous multiplane imaging attempts

Real-time two-dimensional echocardiography was an advance over M-mode, providing more accurate spatial anatomic information about cardiac structures. As summarized recently by Pearlman [17], three-dimensional echocardiography is also likely to provide more accurate quantitative information as to cardiac spatial morphology than is currently available by two-dimensional techniques. One example of this is the work of Eaton [18] where more accurate left ventricular volumes were possible given the ability to acquire more tomographic cuts through the ventricle.

Several methods have been employed to increase spatial information in ultrasonic images. Robinson [12] reconstructed arbitrary two-dimensional planes and three-dimensional images from a series of mutually perpendicular two-dimensional slices stored in a computer. More recently, Geiser [13] used an instrumented mechanical arm attached to a two-dimensional system to relay positional information to a computer for later three-dimensional reconstruction of spatial information about the heart. Moritz and Pearlman [9] published three-dimensional reconstructions of ventricular volumes using a spark gap position sensing system to control the computer-based image processing.

These approaches require a bulky transducer assembly and considerable computer processing time to recreate the three-dimensional image. In each case, the three-dimensional image does not present the original ultrasonic data but the resultant line drawing of cardiac targets such as endocardium that result from complex automated or manual edge detection systems.

Two techniques for acquiring orthogonal images have been reported. Curling [19] showed the feasibility of switching between two arrays in an intra-esophageal assembly for the alternate acquisition of two orthogonal planes. Miwa [20] constructed a system capable of producing orthogonal images by linking the transducers from two B-mode mechanical sector scanners. The cost and transducer ergonomics of these systems, however, limit their widespread use.

Ideally, a three-dimensional ultrasound imaging device would be able to acquire images from multiple planes simultaneously, allowing real-time analysis and presentation of three-dimensional data. Although current systems are capable of images with high line density, wide field of view, and video frame rates, the data acquisition rate limits this performance to a single plane. This occurs because the speed of sound is fixed in tissue, limiting the number of lines that can be displayed per unit of time. Imaging in multiple planes, without parallel processing, can only be achieved by sacrificing one of the image parameters mentioned above, degrading the potential diagnostic utility of the device.

Orthogonal mode imaging

The results of this study indicate that images of the quality currently available in one plane may be created simultaneously in two orthogonal planes from the same hand held transducer. The system is simple enough to be added to an existing ultrasonic scanner and the machine operating characteristics are sufficiently like those of conventional imaging systems to make this technology readily available.

As clinically applied, the size of the current transducer is large enough that skin contact is lost in certain views, such as the apical four chamber. Reduction in the area making contact with the skin is required before easy manipulability can be assured.

Even though clinical experience with this system is still limited, an operator can easily and rapidly obtain a three-dimensional subjective impression of the size, geometry and relationships of cardiac structures not readily possible by conventional single plane techniques. Specific applications of the system for improved diagnostic or quantitative purposes await continued use.

The development of a format appropriate for the simultaneous display of two real-time sectors arcs has been a unique aspect of this project. The two-dimensional projection technique currently strains the ability of the user to interpret all of the ultrasound information presented. From our experience it takes time to adjust to this presentation and an alternate display method may be necessary. The perspective projection method is uniquely simple, however, and may be improved in time.

There are problems with the current O-mode format, the most significant being the transducer geometry. The decreased signal-to-noise ratio due to the bow-tie shaped aperture is a drawback and a more conventional rectangular aperture would be preferable. This would require an $N \times N$ element array, but for the O-mode application it might be multiplexed into rows and columns, simplifying design, construction, and wiring tasks. Such an array has been fabricated and tested and is awaiting hardware implementation into the system.

O-mode is a significant first step toward real-time, three-dimensional imaging. This approach is capable of interrogating a three-dimensional sample volume in real-time from a single phased array transducer. Further improvements in the Explososcan parallel processing system combined with future improvements in transducer design will likely provide more than two simultaneous planes.

Acknowledgments

These data were originally published in Snyder JE, Kisslo J, and von Ramm OT: Real-time orthogonal mode scanning of the Heart. I. System Design. Journal of the American College of Cardiology. 7: 1279–85, 1986.

References

1. Braunwald E: Heart disease. Second Edition, WB Saunders Co, Philadelphia, 1984; 453.
2. Edler I, Hertz CH: The use of ultrasonic reflectoscope for the continuous recording of movements of heart walls. Kungl Fysiograf Sallskap Lund Forh 1954; 24: 1–19.
3. Bom N, Lancee CT, Honkoop J, Hugenholtz PG: Ultrasonic viewer for cross-sectional analysis of moving cardiac structures. Biomed Engng 1971; 6: 500–508.
4. Griffith JM, Henry WL: A sector scanner for real-time two-dimensional echocardiography. Circulation 1974; 49: 1147–1152.
5. Eggleton RC, Feigenbaum H, Johnston KW, Weyman AE, Dillon JC, Chang S: Visualization of cardiac dynamics with a real-time, B-mode ultrasonic scanner. In: White DN (ed) Ultrasound in Medicine. New York, Plenum Press 1975; 1: 385–395.
6. von Ramm OT, Thurstone FL: Cardiac Imaging using a phased array ultrasound system: I. System design. Circulation 1976; 53: 258–262.
7. Kisslo J, von Ramm OT, Thurstone FL: Cardiac Imaging using a phased array ultrasound system: II. Clinical technique and application. Circulation 1976; 53: 262–267.
8. Feigenbaum H: Echocardiography. Fourth Edition, Lea and Febiger, Philadelphia, 1981: 1–46.
9. Moritz WE, Pearlman AS, McCabe DH, Medema DK, Ainsworth ME, Boles MS: An ultrasonic technique for imaging the ventricle in three dimensions and calculating its volume. IEEE Transactions on Biomedical Engineering 1983; 30: 482–492.
10. Nikravesh PE, Skorton DJ, Chandran YM, Attarwala YM, Pandian N, Kerber RE: Computerized three-dimensional finite element reconstruction of the left ventricle from cross-sectional echocardiograms. Ultrasonic Imaging 1984; 6: 48–59.
11. Brinkley JF, Moritz WE, Baker DW: Ultrasonic three-dimensional imaging and volume from a series of arbitrary sector scans. Ultrasound in Medicine and Biology 1978; 4: 317–327.
12. Robinson DE: Display of three-dimensional ultrasonic data for medical diagnosis. J Acoustical Soc Am 1972; 52: 673–687.
13. Geiser EA, Ariet M, Conetta DA, Lupkiewicz SM, Christie LG, Conti CR: Dynamic three-dimensional echocardiographic reconstruction of the intact human left ventricle: Technique and initial observations in patients. Am Heart J 1982; 103: 1056–1065.
14. Shattuck DP, Weinshenker MD, Smith SW, von Ramm OT: Explososcan: A parallel processing technique for high speed ultrasound imaging with linear phased arrays. J Acoustical Soc Am 1984; 75: 1273–1282.
15. von Ramm OT, Weinshenker MD, Snyder JE: High speed echocardiography. Proceedings of the 5th Congress of the European Federation of Societies for Ultrasound in Medicine 1984; 5: 41.
16. Tuy HK, Tuy LT: Direct 2-D display of 3-D images. IEEE Computer Graphics and Applications 1984; 4: 29.
17. Pearlman AS, Moritz WE: Three-dimensional reconstruction of the left ventricle from multiple two-dimensional ultrasonic images. Automedica 1984; 5: 133–149.
18. Eaton LW, Maughan WL, Shoukas AA, Weiss JL: Accurate volume determination in the isolated ejecting canine left ventricle by two-dimensional echocardiography. Circulation 1979; 60: 320–326.
19. Curling PE, Newsome LR, Rogers A, Hillard W, Sutherland J, Martin J, Nagle D, Waller JL: 2D transesophageal echocardiography: A bidirectional phased array probe for temporal monitoring. Anesthesiology 1984; 61: A159.
20. Miwa H, Hayashi H, Shimura T, Murakami K: Simultaneous multifrequency ultrasonography: The principle and technology. IEEE Ultrasonics Symposium 1981; 655–659.

Index of subjects